**Issues in Midw**

*For Churchill Livingstone*

*Commissioning editor:* Mary Law
*Project editor:* Dinah Thom
*Project manager:* Neil A. Dickson
*Project controller:* Nicola S. Haig
*Copy editor:* Teresa Brady
*Design direction:* Judith Wright
*Sales promotion executive:* Hilary Brown

# Issues in Midwifery

Edited by

**Tricia Murphy-Black** MSc PhD RGN RM
Research and Development Adviser, Simpson Memorial Maternity Pavilion,
Edinburgh, UK

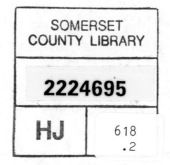

CHURCHILL LIVINGSTONE
EDINBURGH HONG KONG LONDON MADRID MELBOURNE NEW YORK AND
TOKYO 1995

CHURCHILL LIVINGSTONE
Medical Division of Longman Group Limited

Distributed in the United States of America by Churchill
Livingstone Inc., 650 Avenue of the Americas, New York,
N.Y. 10011, and by associated companies, branches and
representatives throughout the world.

© Longman Group Limited 1995

First published 1995

ISBN 0 443 04864 9

**British Library Cataloguing in Publication Data**
A catalogue record for this book is available from the
British Library.

**Library of Congress Cataloging in Publication Data**
Issues in midwifery / edited by Tricia Murphy-Black.
          p.      cm.
   Includes index.
   ISBN 0-443-04864-9
   1. Midwives. I. Murphy-Black, Tricia.
   [DNLM: 1. Midwifery. WQ 160 I86 1995]
RG950.I86 1995
362. 1'982--dc20
DNLM/DLC
for Library of Congress                                    94-29342

120164 7 104566 1

The
publisher's
policy is to use
paper manufactured
from sustainable forests

Produced through Longman Malaysia, TCP.

# Contents

# Contributors

**Joanne Alexander** PhD RGN RM MTD FPCert
Principal Lecturer in Midwifery, University of Portsmouth, UK

**Lesley Barclay** RN CM BA MEd
Professor of Nursing in Family Health, University of Technology, Sydney and Southern Sydney Area Service, Australia

**Sharon Cochrane** RGN RM ADM
Midwife, Labour Ward, University College Hospital, London, UK

**Joan Donley** OBE RN RMN RM
Domiciliary Midwife, Auckland, New Zealand

**Valerie E. M. Fleming** RGON RM MA
Lecturer in Midwifery, Department of Nursing and Midwifery, Massey University, Palmerston North, New Zealand

**Sheila Harvey** RN SCM MN
Co-ordinator, Nurse-Midwifery Programme, Foothills Hospital, Calgary, Alberta; Adjunct Assistant Professor, University of Calgary, Calgary, Alberta, Canada

**Judy Hedwig**
Midwife, Palmerston North, New Zealand

**Kate Hughes** LLB
Vancouver, British Columbia, Canada

**Kate Isherwood** BSc(Hons) PhD RGN RM ADM
Integrated Midwife, Pembrokeshire, West Wales, UK

**Rosemary Jenkins** RN RM MTD DMS MBIM
Formerly Director of Professional Affairs, Royal College of Midwives, UK

**Karyn J. Kaufman** BSN MS DrPH
Chair, Midwifery Education Programme; Associate Professor,
Faculty of Health Sciences, McMaster University, Hamilton,
Ontario, Canada

**Maggie Lecky-Thompson** RN RM ACMI Accred DipHerbMed
National Representative, Australian Society of Independent
Midwives, Australia

**Christine Midgley** MEd RGN RM MTD
Course Director, Pre-Registration Midwifery, Birmingham and
Solihull College of Nursing and Midwifery, Birmingham, UK

**Tricia Murphy-Black** MSc PhD RGN RM
Research and Development Adviser, Simpson Memorial
Maternity Pavilion, Edinburgh, UK

**Anne Nixon** RM HonBA
Faculty French Stream, Laurentian University Midwifery
Programme, Sudbury, Ontario, Canada

**J. Alison Rice** BSN MS RN SCM
Assistant Professor, University of British Columbia, School of
Nursing, Vancouver, British Columbia, Canada

**Joyce Roberts** CNM PhD FAAN FACNM
Professor and Head, Department of Maternal-Child Nursing,
College of Nursing, University of Illinois at Chicago; Clinical
Chief, Parent/Child Health Division, University of Illinois
Hospital, University of Illinois at Chicago, USA

**M. Sheelagh Scattergood** BA RGN RM MTD BTA
Senior Midwife Teacher, Bolton and Salford College of
Midwifery and Nursing, Bolton UK

**Holliday Tyson** SCM MHSc
Director, Laurentian University Midwifery Programme,
Sudbury, Ontario, Canada

**Arlene Vandersloot** RM
Clinical Teacher, Laurentian University, Sudbury, Ontario,
Canada

# Preface

Midwifery is facing many exciting challenges at a time of ever increasing demands that health care be efficient, effective and equitable. Midwives have had a long struggle to have their services recognised and in a number of countries, it is the consumer who has provided the impetus required for midwives to assert their position in providing care for women undergoing a normal physiological event.

Maternity services are changing in the UK, with the impetus of government reports which place the woman and her baby at the centre of care. Canada is at a pivotal point, with the legalistion of midwifery in a number of provinces; midwives have the opportunity and challenge to start with services which are not weighed down by tradition. Australian and New Zealand midwives also face enormous change in their systems and recognise that this is the time for the midwife to emerge from the apron strings of nursing. The US is also appreciating that midwifery has something to offer; something which may be valued more within their changing health care systems.

The three main sections in this book, independent midwifery, the education of midwives and models both of and for midwifery, are addressed by authors from a variety of countries and different health care systems. The differences in the approaches, as well as the similarities, provide an opportunity to learn from others. The interpretation of the section titles varies: independent midwifery within the UK describes the work of independent midwives, while Australian and New Zealand authors address the issue of independence of midwifery. The establishment of graduate education for midwives in these countries prompts a range of views of the educational system and the position of midwives. Perhaps it is graduate education that will thrust midwives into the professional arena with the confidence and assertiveness required.

There are four chapters which address issues not easily cate-gorised with others: concerned with politics, relationships be-tween doctors, nurses and midwives, and the impact of male dominance on a service for women. The chapter on the impact of HIV asks difficult questions of a profession that has not yet had to deal with the problem on a large scale in the UK.

If this book has midwives agreeing with all of it, then it has failed. If midwives debate and argue about its content, it is hoped that a greater understanding of the challenges we face will emerge. If so, the result will help to meet the aim of all midwives: that the outcomes of midwifery care are a healthy and happy mother and baby.

Edinburgh, 1995                                                           T. M-B.

# Midwifery – a matter of politics

*Rosemary Jenkins*

## INTRODUCTION

Midwives do not enter politics – or at least this would seem to be the case at present in the United Kingdom. There are no midwives, as there are lawyers, doctors, teachers, civil servants or nurses, in the British Parliament, either in the House of Commons or the House of Lords.

However, this assumes a narrow definition of politics, encompassing only those activities directly concerned with the legislative process. Politics is broader than this. In its widest sense it concerns the way a society is governed or controlled, the systems, which are in place within a society, the decisions made within these systems, which serve to control the society, and the impact of those decisions upon the people. It also concerns the actions of people, as individuals or groups which are directed at influencing the existing order of society. Politics is about the systems that exist within a society; it is about local as well as national government, and it is about the people, who, as individuals or in pressure groups, fight either to change the systems or to retain the status quo. Above all it is about taking action to influence the way society is organised or about the way people are organised within it.

## WHAT POLITICAL ISSUES SHOULD CONCERN MIDWIVES?

### Health care systems

Although independent and lay midwives, in small numbers, practise in many countries, the great majority of midwives work within the prevailing health care systems. Their work, the way they are able to practise and the mechanisms they can use to influence their work environment can be heavily dependent upon the system in which they work, and most of these systems are politically driven.

Health care provision and the method of financing health care are invariably determined by a country's legislature and commonly reflect the political bias of the government. These biases fall along a political spectrum which runs from the extreme of centralised command, as in the pre-1990 USSR, to minimalist government as seen in the USA, particularly under Republican administrations. In the United Kingdom (UK), Clement Attlee's radical left government of 1945–1951 contrasted with the radical right government of Margaret Thatcher.

Health care provision under these four political systems shows the same spectrum of bias.

#### Health care in the USA

Government funding of health care in the USA is confined to providing a minimal 'safety net' through its Medicaid and Medicare systems, for the poor and the old. People are expected to fund their own health care costs through private insurance although this is often provided as part of an employment benefit. This link with employment effectively excludes the unemployed from such benefits, and even the state schemes are not open-ended.

The results of this minimal approach to health care are varied. For those who can pay, the American hospital system can be one of the best in the world. It is customer-oriented, and provides levels of hotel services which can only be matched in the private systems of other countries. However, the uncontrolled reimbursement of medical treatment has the potential to lead to overdiagnosis and overtreatment. Conversely, it is estimated that many millions of Americans are currently not covered for medical costs either from the state schemes or private insurance. The negative impact of this upon the maternity services is seen in the poor rate of infant mortality in the USA: 10.1/1000 compared, for example, with Denmark's 7.3/1000 (World Health Organization 1992).

However the lack of tight central control allows for local innovation and initiatives that can bring positive change. Health services dependent upon prepaid insurance, or 'health maintenance organizations', are now increasingly common. The financial success of these groups depends as much upon preventing ill health, and therefore containing health care costs, as it does on providing effective rather than excessive health care. Similarly, the lack of central legislative control does enable, in a country not noted for any strength in the midwifery profession, the continued practice of lay midwifery.

### The health care system in the former Soviet Union

The system in the former Soviet Union (FSU) could not be more different. All decisions about health care, including the available money, the training and use of different staff grades and the provision of hospital beds, were made centrally and filtered through to state, regional, city and hospital level.

The system, like the FSU is bankrupt, and conclusions should not be drawn based upon the lack of financing. Constitutionally, all people within the FSU have the right to health care. The system is also very uniform, based upon hospital, polyclinic (outpatient) and dispensary (local clinic) provision.

There is however little accountability towards the users of the system, rather the accountability is to the State. Thus for example, copious statistics on health service activity are processed centrally, yet there is little will or pressure to change outmoded care. Mistakes made in central direction are also magnified as they are passed through to service level. Marked examples, of this are the overprovision of doctors, most of whom are underpaid and undervalued, and the underprovision and undervaluing of middle grade health professionals, such as midwives.

### The UK National Health Service until the 1980s

The UK National Health Service (NHS), as envisaged in 1948, embodied the principles of the central command mechanism, although it did not abolish the right of people to receive, and professionals to practise, private health care. Neither, in 1948 did it provide for universal health care under one system, as the health service (hospital and practitioner services) and the local authority (community and ambulance services) remained separate until the NHS Reorganisation Act 1973. It did however seek to ensure universal provision and equity of access.

What the National Health Service singularly failed to do was to provide variety of health care to meet the diversity of health care need. It has consistently remained dominated by the hospital sector, financially supportive of acute rather than primary care and driven by the agenda of a powerful medical profession.

### The National Health Service at present

A shift to a more radical right-wing ideology in the 1980s eventually led to a review of the NHS. A White Paper (preceding the publication of a Bill to reform the National Health Service) was published in 1989. *Working for Patients* (Department of Health 1989) heralded the most comprehensive reform of UK health care since 1948.

The chain of command between hospitals and other health services and central government was to be broken, thus allowing all those providing health care (commonly referred to as 'providers') to manage themselves by applying for and becoming 'NHS Trusts'. Subject only to broad central direction, these providers of health care would be able to exercise autonomy in decisions on how to provide health care.

The second, and equally important change was the introduction of a limited, internal market for health care. Hospitals would no longer receive their share of the health care money automatically. District Health Authorities and Boards (commonly referred to as 'purchasers') would in future receive government allocations to enable them to buy whatever health care they assessed would be necessary to meet the health care needs of the population they served. It would be open to them to purchase these services from whichever 'provider unit' they wished, thus placing the providers in direct competition with each other. Competition, it was argued would introduce a pressure upon the providers to offer better services, at the same time as keeping the costs for services as low as possible. The money available to providers to run their services would be dependent upon how successful they might be in obtaining contracts for these services from the DHAs.

## Rationing of health care

The above four examples demonstrate that the way in which any government chooses to deliver health care to its population will depend largely upon the political bias of the government. There is however one underlying problem that faces all governments, and all health care systems: there is never enough money in the system to meet all the demands upon it. The patchy provision of care in the UK, prior to 1948, was not dissimilar to the same patchy distribution in the United States today, with large numbers effectively excluded from receiving care. The hope that centrally provided care, paid for by taxation, would treat current ill health and then lead to a diminished need for services was a fallacy in 1948, and continues to be so today. Whether taxation (the UK), private insurance (USA) or earmarked social insurance (the Netherlands) is the mode of funding, all systems have to develop rationing mechanisms.

The need to do this has become particularly acute during the past quarter-century. The supply of health care has become more expensive through developing technologies and techniques, and the demand has also risen, fuelled by increasing expectations and demographic trends. The percentage of the very elderly is rising, and with this the disproportionate demand their needs generate.

Maternity services cannot be separated out from the three questions that are currently being asked of health care: what should be provided; how should it be provided, and how should it be financed? Indeed there may be reasons why these questions are being asked first of maternity care than of many other specialities. The main receivers of care are fit, young women who are experiencing a normal life event; the use of the skills of doctors may be an expensive means of giving care, and there are other health professionals whose training may be more appropriate to meet the needs of this group – midwives.

The debate is growing on how to make explicit choices in health care provision. In the state of Oregon, USA, the health service authorities, using public participation and consultation, have defined a list of those treatments that will be financed by Medicaid (Health Services Commission 1991). In the Netherlands, a government Committee on Choices in Health Care (Dunning 1992) has just published its report. It suggests the adoption of a more rational approach to the determination of what health care should be provided by the social insurance mechanism. By implication, making choices about the health care to be provided also means making choices about the health care not to be provided.

### Midwives' role in a changing system

Midwives' cannot ignore these political pressures. As centrally controlled health care systems give way, as has happened in the United Kingdom, new flexibility will enable health care planners and managers to seek new ways to provide cost-effective health care and, increasingly, to decide what care should be provided given a finite income.

Changing the face of maternity care to meet this new agenda will challenge the existing order and existing hierachies, and has the potential to become a political 'struggle' between policy makers and medical staff. Arguments about the cost-effectiveness of midwifery-based, primary focused maternity care may lead to direct conflict with the other main protagonists: general practitioners and obstetricians. Midwives can remain passive, becoming pawns in this struggle, or can begin to play an active part in determining their role in the changing pattern of health care and maternity care in particular.

## The politics of gender

There can hardly be an activity more rooted in the feminine world than the practice of midwifery. Its development is traditional and global. It started as the wise woman of the village, the helper who would support and 'mother' the woman in childbirth. The skills passed from generation to generation are not the product of a modern medical system, but of a social support system, acknowledged and demanded by women through time and across geographical boundaries. As such it is possible to interpret the history and position of midwives, vicariously, as the history and position of women generally.

The historical achievements of midwives are largely unrecorded. As women they were unlikely to have access to the education that would enable them to write about their work.

### Control of midwifery

Control mechanisms, first the Church and then the emerging

medical profession, comprised men who effectively ensured that midwifery remained in a subservient position. The doctor, practising obstetrics and offering his services to the rich and influential, eclipsed the midwife of the 19th century, remembered only for her Sarah Gamp image.

Yet in the United Kingdom there seemed to be a positive reversal of this situation. After over 20 years of campaigning, midwifery was recognised in statute and a training required for the right to practise. It would be wrong to trivialise this important milestone but the struggle to bring the 1902 Midwives' Act to the statute book resulted in compromises that perpetuated the medical (male) dominance of midwifery for most of the 20th century. It was not until the 1970s that the chairmanship of the statutory body, the Central Midwives' Board, passed to a midwife.

A system of supervision of midwives by local medical officers of health was set up in 1936. These medical officers were charged with overseeing the standards and worthiness of the practising midwives. They were not required to do the work involved. Non-medical supervisors of midwives (women) performed the supervisory visits, wrote the reports and advised the midwives. Even this division of labour mirrored that which commonly prevails between man's work and woman's work, the man's being supervisory and high status, the woman's task-oriented and of lower status. The medical supervisor of midwives position was only discontinued with the 1974 NHS Reorganisation Act.

## The nature and organisation of midwifery

It is not only in the control of midwifery that gender conflict arises, but also in the nature of the work and in comparisons with the nature of medical practice. Midwifery is expectant and supportive. The traditional practice has been to enable women to labour and give birth, not to intervene in the process. Active intervention is the domain of the doctor.

Other subtle aspects of midwifery suggest a feminine organisation. The tight hierarchy and patronage displayed by the medical and other professions is not in evidence. The flattened structure of the supervision of midwifery is jealously guarded. When, in 1988, a hierarchical structure comprising seven clinical grades was introduced to midwifery as well as nursing, midwives then, as now, decried the grading levels as 'not fitting' the practice of midwifery.

Even the traditional means of training by the apprenticeship and mentor system, with skills passed from midwife to midwife rather than through formal theoretical learning, is much more a feminine idea.

Thus far, that midwifery is traditionally organised along feminine lines has not benefited either the status or payment of the midwife. All female-dominated occupations are consistently underpaid and undervalued. The sharp contrast between midwifery and dentistry underlines this. Both occupations, unlike that of the doctor, are highly specific in their nature, one tending pregnancy, the other tending teeth. A university-based 5-year training is required for dentistry, a 3-year middle grade training for midwifery. The subsequent status and pay of each show the same wide variation. Either one is overvalued or the other undervalued. What is indisputable is that one is traditionally carried out by men the other is a female occupation, serving women. However the latter part of the 20th century has witnessed a strong feminist movement, and discrimination on grounds of sex is now unlawful.

## Women's demand for non-interventionist care

Although equality of opportunity is still a long way off there are signs that women are becoming more assertive and this is becoming clear in maternity care. The ascendancy of man over woman, doctor over woman, doctor over midwife reached its height in the mid-1970s in the United Kingdom. The induction of labour had become almost commonplace, with 50–60% of labours medically induced in some hospital units. Home delivery had almost disappeared as an alternative to the consultant-led hospital. Midwifery was in danger of being reclassified as obstetric nursing, with many midwives acting as doctor's assistants rather than fulfilling their own autonomous role. It was women, the users of the service, who demonstrated publicly outside the Royal Free Hospital in London, and called into question the prevailing obstetric practices. Particularly in the United Kingdom, this political protest was taken up by consumer groups who began the long campaign for greater balance in maternity care provision.

In 1991 the Select Committee on Health of the British Parliament announced a major investigation into the provision of maternity care, to focus particularly upon the needs of women for whom there were no complications. Select Committees work on the basis of calling for evidence from any interested party, analysing the evidence and producing a report based on the evidence. The report of the Select Committee was published in March 1992 (Select Committee on Health 1992). Through their representative groups, and as individuals, many women chose to give evidence to the Committee. They gave three overwhelming messages: they wanted continuity of carer, particularly to know their caregiver during their labour; they wanted choice in the care they could receive and they wanted control over the process of childbirth. In Victoria, Australia, 12 000 miles away, a similar investigation had revealed the same messages (State of Victoria Health Department 1990) (see Ch. 3). As users of systems that had become highly mechanised, highly directed, centralised and dominated by obstetricians, these women were finally demanding a return to the expectant, enabling and supportive female-oriented care traditionally provided by midwives.

## The politics of poverty

The impact of poverty and social deprivation upon health expectancy is well recognised. Perinatal and infant mortality rates show vast intercountry variation, interregional variation within countries and variation between social classes. In 1984 in the United Kingdom, the stillbirth rate for social class I was half that of social class V (4/1000 and 8/1000). The perinatal mortality rates for East Birmingham and Peterborough were 12.2/1000 and 6.6/1000 (Office of Population Census and Surveys 1990). These variations are so great that it is probable that improvements in the living standards of women and their families could result in the single largest improvement in pregnancy outcome, and it is now being recognised that to target professional help at these groups will reap benefits. In the document of the Royal College of Midwives (RCM) *Towards a Healthy Nation* (Royal College of Midwives 1991) it was stated: 'There are indications that the maternity services need to give greater priority to target at-risk groups in order to reduce further perinatal mortality and morbidity'.

Professionally, midwives are now recognising the significance of tailoring support to socially disadvantaged women, of increasing antenatal support and of assisting women, for example, who wish to stop smoking. However, the final section of this chapter will argue that midwives have not taken a strong political stand in order to influence government policy towards those who are poor.

## Environmental politics

The first ever World Summit on the environment was held in 1992 in Rio de Janiero. Although the reasons for and solutions to many specific environmental issues lack consensus support, there is general agreement that the profligate use of resources should stop. Developing countries particularly have drawn attention to the disproportionate use of resources by the developed world. This environmental argument could be used powerfully in support of increasing the work of midwives, with their low technology approach to helping women.

Compare the purchase costs of a Pinards stethoscope with that of an electronic fetal heart monitor. Furthermore, the former needs no subsequent maintenance. In a large study in Dublin (MacDonald et al 1985) it was shown that there was minimal difference between two randomly assigned groups of women, one monitored with a fetal stethoscope, the other with continuous monitoring, and that the difference had disappeared when the children were followed up 1 year later. Yet the use of electronic fetal monitoring remains widespread in developed countries.

Midwifery, dependent as it is upon expectant and supportive care is 'ecologically sound' yet can achieve results comparable to care dependent upon the use of expensive technology.

## Political issues and the midwife's role in them

The four strands of potential political activity identified here, namely health care systems, gender, poverty and the environment, should not be seen in isolation from each other. How the world's resources can be used efficiently is not too different a question from 'how can available health care resources be used efficiently?' Achieving equity for women and equity for the poor will have many of the same solutions. Indeed women make up a disproportionate number of poor.

What is true of these problems is that increasing the role of midwives would make a positive, albeit small, contribution to some of the solutions. It is also true that to reorient maternity care along noninterventionist lines requires more than just small scale local effort, but needs a political will to change. The next section debates whether midwives have that will.

## ARE MIDWIVES POTENTIAL POLITICAL ACTIVISTS?

The introduction to this chapter suggested that political activity could take place inside the system (by becoming a member of Parliament or a local councillor), by working actively within a politically determined system (for example a health service) or by attempting to influence from the outside (by being a member of a pressure group). There is a broad political agenda facing midwifery and the maternity services, and yet evidence that midwives are responding politically remains very weak. There is no midwife in the British Parliament. There are very few midwives who have reached positions of broad influence within the Health Service, as general managers for example.

Perhaps the essential strengths of the midwife militate against her becoming politically active. The midwife will usually be a woman (notwithstanding the few men who take up the career). She will be choosing a woman-centred occupation and one that is very firmly wedded to the development of close personal relationships, that is, with the woman and her family. The nature of midwifery is that it takes a secondary role (or it should) in the childbirth process, supporting and enabling rather than leading in the activity. It may be that the people attracted to the profession, and best able to function as midwives, are the people least able to take political action, least able to assert their own view over the views of others and least able to negotiate from a position of strength.

There is also little past evidence that even when there is the opportunity to use the collective will of midwifery, through the use of a professional organisation, that midwives use this channel to make political points. In the past 10 years only six resolutions of the Royal College of Midwives branch delegates' meetings have addressed issues related to poverty; four have been specifically on maternity grants, one on child care facilities and one only on general welfare benefits.

There are however some notable and very powerful exceptions to this. An early example was the eventual passing of the 1902 Midwives' Act in England and Wales. A small group of midwives, banded together in the Midwives' Institute (later to become the Royal College of Midwives), negotiated and debated for 20 years with politicians, and against a strong medical lobby, to bring the Act onto the statute book. It was not done for the benefit of the midwife but to ensure the availability of trained assistance at childbirth to all women regardless of their means. The task seemed almost impossible particularly as very few politicians would even discuss matters relating to midwifery. It was not considered fit for polite conversation and was anyway of interest only to women, not to politicians.

Much more recently there have been examples, particularly when an issue has threatened midwifery. In 1986 the United Kingdom Central Council for Nursing, Midwifery and Health Visiting (UKCC) published a major consultation document on future education for nurses, midwives and health visitors. *Project 2000* (United Kingdom Central Council 1986) suggested a future diploma level training based upon a 2-year foundation course in health studies, followed by specific training for the branch of nursing chosen by the student. There were to be five branches, the adult, the child, mental handicap, mental illness and midwifery. There was a national outcry from UK midwives who, through a large consultation exercise led by the Royal College of Midwives, indicated clearly their separate professional status and their view that if there were to be a diploma course it should be a 3-year, separate, and direct entry training. The UKCC acquiesced and with money made available from the Department of Health preregistration midwifery training was re-established. Midwifery was withdrawn as a branch of nursing.

At opposite ends of the world unlicensed midwives have succeeded in achieving licensure, like the British experience, against fierce medical opposition. Midwives now have the right to practise in New Zealand on a par with their medical colleagues. Like general practitioners, they can set up in practice, practise autonomously and their pay and status are similar. This struggle is described more fully in Chapter 4.

Lay midwives in the state of Ontario, Canada were challenged by doctors, and when one attended a woman who had a stillbirth, the medical profession brought a court case against her with the aim of making midwifery illegal. The midwives in Ontario so organised themselves that instead of making midwifery illegal, the judge advised that midwives should be legally recognised and licensed. Midwifery training in Ontario has been established.

In Western Germany an old law on the statute book required a midwife to be present at all births. Germany has a preponderance of obstetricians, most of whom performed the deliveries with the midwife in assistance. When the obstetricians approached the German Government to have the law repealed, German midwives organised in opposition to this move and won. The law remains (Wagner M, personal communication).

Midwifery in Romania was abolished in 1978 by the Ceaucescu regime. Practising midwives lost their jobs and training was withdrawn. From that time young women entered maternity units after limited education and 'hygiene' studies. A workshop for these women, the first time they had met together, was held under the direction of the World Health Organization and UNICEF in 1992. They were asked for their initial assessment of what they needed if midwifery was to become a strong profession again. Their first priority was to form an association so that they could begin to discuss and bring pressure upon the authorities so that midwifery could again be recognised. They saw clearly the need to exercise the collective will (Jenkins 1992).

## WHERE ARE THE OPPORTUNITIES TO INFLUENCE POLITICAL DECISIONS AND THEIR IMPACT?

### Importance of organisation

From the examples of the last section, it would appear that success in influencing the political decision making processes lies in strong organisation. Certainly when there is a single issue on which to campaign, working together as a group does have advantages. However, the formula for success is not as simple as this. There are many examples where midwives' organisations exist, yet midwifery remains weak within the health care system.

This could be particularly true of the Royal College of Midwives. During the 1970s midwifery became almost extinct as an autonomous profession yet in 1981 the RCM celebrated its 100th year. It represented up to 80% of the midwives in the United Kingdom yet it was possible for the profession to accept, albeit unwillingly in many quarters, the Nurses', Midwives' and Health Visitors' Act, abolishing the separate statutory body (Central Midwives' Board) so keenly fought for just 100 years before. (A number of statutory bodies were combined in the United Kingdom Central Council for Nursing, Midwifery and Health Visiting (UKCC).) Important concessions were achieved (the Midwifery Committees at UKCC and National Board level) but generally in spite of an apparent collectivism, ground was being lost.

The 1970s also saw the almost complete demise of direct entry training for midwives – the training that set them apart from the nurse. Some midwives were so dissatisfied with this situation that a breakaway group, the Association of Radical Midwives (ARM), was formed, with the aim of returning back to the roots of midwifery practice.

Usually a split in a campaign's ranks will weaken its overall results. There were, however, certain points about this particular split that may have strengthened rather than weakened the growing demand from midwives that they should be able to practise autonomously. First, most of those midwives who joined the ARM continued their membership of the RCM. Secondly and importantly, both organisations were pursuing the same goal even though they were taking different paths towards it. As the radical arm of midwifery, ARM could continue to be challenging and stand aside from the accepted establishment. The RCM, on the other hand continued to rely upon having the political doors open to it, in order to influence from the inside, but had to do so by appearing conciliatory and in favour of the established wisdom. Fortuitously rather than by design, the British midwives found a complementary formula that began to work in order to bring about change. Then, as now, it relied upon good communication between the two organisations (not always easy in the beginning).

The RCM also began to devise new political strategies in order to increase its influence. In 1985 its Council approved the establishment of a press, parliamentary and publicity section and employed an officer to work in this area.

## Influencing change at national level

The willingness to use the political channels open to them, and to seek professional advice to do so, has enabled midwives in the UK to be part of an experimental reorientation of health care on a scale not seen since the establishment in the 19th century of the medical profession as the key health workers.

Influenced not only by the evidence of women, but by the evidence submitted to it by the RCM, the Select Committee on Health recommended a complete reappraisal of the British maternity services. Concerning midwives, the Select Committee (1992) recommended:

That the status of midwives as professionals is acknowledged in their terms and conditions of employment which should be based on the presumption that they have a right to develop and audit their own professional standards;

that we should move as rapidly as possible towards a situation in which midwives have their own caseload, and take full responsibility for the women who are under their care;

that midwives should be given the opportunity to establish and run midwife managed maternity units within and outside hospitals;

that the right of midwives to admit women to NHS hospitals should be made explicit.

In the UK parliamentary system, a Select Committee does not have the force of government although the Government is obliged to respond to any recommendations within 2 months. The Government response, when it came, was vilified by a number of midwives who had hoped for a complete acceptance of all the Committee's recommendations. However, the response did not reject the findings of the Committee, rather it proposed further examination of the way maternity should be organised in the UK. An 'Expert Group' chaired by a Health Minister undertook this task. Their report *Changing Childbirth* has recommended a radical revision of maternity services in England.

## Change at local level

Whilst it is essential to pursue change at national level it is equally important to demand alternative systems at a local level. The first section of this chapter discussed the recent changes in the National Health Service in the United Kingdom, and mentioned both the increased local flexibility that this has brought and the 'internal market' comprising purchasers of health care as well as providers. There are ways in which these innovations can also be used to effect change.

The purchasers of health care (District Health Authorities/ Boards) are charged with drawing up contracts for health care that will meet the needs of the population they cover. These contracts are still in their infancy as the NHS changes were only introduced in April 1991, following the implementation of the National Health Service and Community Care Act 1990. Gradually these contracts are becoming more explicit rather than being merely 'block' statements about the service to be purchased and the price to be paid for it; they are beginning to stipulate the detail of services to be provided and the standard of those services.

It is likely that this contractual mechanism will in the future hold a real opportunity to require of providers to change the service they offer, particularly to meet the requirements of users of the services. Important to this process will be the general managers, chairmen, directors of purchasing and directors of public health of the authorities. If midwives have a will to change the system, they will need to supplement the national activities of their organisations by building alliances with these main 'players' in health service provision. They will also need to recognise the difficulties that have always faced women when beginning to assert their needs and views; that these players have themselves usually progressed through the male-dominated and male-devised hierarchies in order to reach the position they occupy. Political activity can be very tortuous.

## Potential allies

Whilst midwives seeking to grasp opportunities to influence political change will constantly meet difficulties, they should also recognise that there are natural alliances which they should develop. The most powerful of these allies, perversely, are the women they serve. Perversely, because women are traditionally weak, but in expressing their demands for change to maternity care they also have become organised and vociferous.

They are also now consulted by policy makers. The government Expert Group which examined maternity care in the wake of the Select Committee Report had four user representatives. They are considered experts. It is also their views which will guide, in time, health authorities in their contract decisions. Patient choice, mediated by expert management of the resources available for health care provision, could become the most powerful factor in the health service.

Midwives could use this force to regain their true position in a way not easy to achieve in the past. They must however listen to what their potential allies are asking for. They will only achieve the changes they seek if they meet the needs of women completely, that is reject the medicalised care model and take again the traditional role as close confidante and supporter of women in childbirth.

Achieving political change also requires the protagonists to examine their own roles and adapt where necessary.

## CONCLUSION

Amongst midwives thee is a nascent sense that they are beginning to achieve recognition of their value. Worldwide, even against organised opposition, they are achieving legal status, the rights to practise and to recognised education programmes. They are beginning to use the power of collective and organised force to effect change for themselves. Some are beginning to see that they can also affect the maternity care systems in which they work, by influencing decisions on staffing levels and grades and on the appropriate technologies to use. Others are directing their influence to national level decision making. There is now little question in the collective mind of the profession about its role in advocating and achieving change in maternity care.

There are however other areas in the political arena into which midwives have scarcely ventured. They are one of the most overtly female groupings worldwide, yet rarely support broad women's issues even on health matters. Women's life expectancy exceeds that of men. In the Netherlands they have a life expectancy at birth of 80 years, while men have only 73 years. But their health expectancy is worse, with women expecting only 58 healthy years, and men 59 (Dunning 1992). There has been no outcry from midwives, on behalf of women, for the reorientation of general health services to redress these imbalances.

Despite laws against sex discrimination and legislation for equal opportunities, women continue to hold low status, low paid employment with little material aid towards child care facilities. They continue to combine this with full household duties, unable to stop work because family finances depend upon their salaries. They continue to be found disproportionately in part-time and poorly protected jobs. Indeed, some midwives will fall into these categories. Yet the collective voice of midwives is rarely raised effectively in support of real change in conditions for women.

As primary workers, midwives throughout the world must daily meet people who are underprivileged, socially deprived and poor. They must also in their work see the deep divisions between the rich and poor. In some parts of the world they must see the devastation wrought upon the environment by uncontrolled industrialisation, and the hurt this brings to families when babies are born damaged by the effects of ecological despoliation. They must witness daily the loss of children, mainly because of poverty, and the deaths of young women which could be averted if those women had access to basic education, family planning methods and good primary health care.

The efforts of individual midwives to alleviate some of these problems are immense, but as a group midwives have thus far failed to raise the collective voice of protest.

Midwives have learned that it is possible, given the will to do so, to change systems, even when the system is entrenched in tradition and subject to powerful vested interests. Their lack of activity on broader political fronts may be due to the vast energy they are still using in order to alter maternity care. The time must now be due when they should be using their new-found political skills, on national and global scales, to plead for all women who are disadvantaged and all families who are poor.

REFERENCES

Department of Health 1989 Working for patients. HMSO, London
Department of Health 1993 Changing childbirth. Part I. Report of the Expert Maternity Group. HMSO, London
Dunning A J 1992 Choices in health care. A report by the Government Committee on Choices in Health Care. The Netherlands Ministry of Welfare, Health and Cultural Affairs, The Hague
Health Services Commission 1991 Oregon Report. Oregon
Jenkins E R 1992 Report of a visit to Romania, prepared for the World Health Organization. Unpublished
MacDonald D, Grant A, Sheridan-Pereira M, Boylan P, Chalmers I 1985 The Dublin randomized controlled trial of intrapartum fetal heart rate monitoring. American Journal of Obstetrics and Gynecology 152: 524–539
Office of Population Census and Surveys 1991 DH3 92/1 Infant and perinatal mortality 1991: RHAs and DHAs. OPCS, London
Royal College of Midwives 1991 Towards a healthy nation. RCM, London
Select Committee on Health 1992 Second Report Maternity Services Session 1991–1992. HMSO, London
State of Victoria Health Department 1990 Having a baby in Victoria. Final report of a ministerial review of birthing services in Victoria, Lumley J (Chair). Health Department, Victoria, Australia.
United Kingdom Central Council for Nursing, Midwifery and Health Visiting 1986 Project 2000: a new preparation for practice. UKCC London
Wagner M 1992 Personal communication
World Health Organization 1992 World Health Statistics Annual 1991. WHO, Geneva

# Independent midwifery

SECTION CONTENTS

# Independent midwifery in the United Kingdom

*Kate Isherwood*

## INTRODUCTION

This chapter looks at independent midwifery in the United Kingdom, that is, at midwives who practise outside the National Health Service to offer continuity of care on an individual basis, charging a fee for their services. Although there are very small numbers of independent midwives, their existence has important implications for the midwifery profession and for the maternity services. To understand better the current situation in the profession, developments during this century are first explored. The rise of independent midwifery in the 1980s and the reasons given for practising independently are discussed next. Personal experiences of some midwives and clients are then described, based on studies of independent midwifery in the UK. The influence of independent midwifery on the profession, and the implications for the future of the maternity services are then considered.

# THE DEVELOPMENT OF MIDWIFERY IN THE 20TH CENTURY

The Midwives' Act reached the statute books in 1902 in England and Wales (1915 in Scotland), and was designed to protect the public from unqualified practitioners (Robinson 1990). Thus the training and registration of midwives began to be regulated in Britain. Local supervising authorities (LSAs), accountable to the Central Midwives' Board (CMB), were set up to supervise midwifery, and had the power to suspend midwives from practice. Inspectors of Midwives were appointed by LSAs to ensure that minimum standards of hygiene and safe practice were met. At that time most midwives, many of them illiterate, were self-employed, receiving payment for service from their clients. Having to pay a fee of 10 shillings to register with the CMB was beyond the means of many. By the 1870s, midwives' fees averaged 7 shillings per delivery. Even by the 1920s, midwives' annual earnings could be as low as £30 (Towler & Bramall 1986).

Under the 1918 Maternal and Child Welfare Act, free state antenatal care became available (but not mandatory) at some local authority clinics. Although the proportion of qualified practising midwives increased from 30% in 1905 to 74% in 1915 (Robinson 1990), many women preferred the unqualified 'handywoman' to a qualified midwife. The handywoman was cheaper, willing to follow local customs and give domestic support (Donnison 1977, Dingwall et al 1988). Under the 1902 Midwives' Act unqualified handywomen could attend women in childbirth under a doctor's supervision; clients and doctors colluded to perpetuate the existence of handywomen until the 1930s (Dingwall et al 1988).

During the 1920s, 50–60% of women were attended in childbirth by only a midwife (Robinson 1990), but in an emergency the midwife had to call a doctor. Services were concentrated around delivery and puerperium, but 80% of pregnant women did receive antenatal care by 1935, either from their own general practitioners (GPs), independent (private) midwives or from local authority midwives at municipal clinics (Towler & Bramall 1986).

## The threat to independent midwifery practice

By the 1930s working conditions were difficult for independent midwives, who constituted nearly 50% of all those in practice

(Donnison 1977). Independent midwifery was threatened by the subsidised local authority clinics and by the rise in hospital births; 36% in 1937 (Robinson 1990). A national salaried midwifery service was proposed to improve the working conditions of midwives and the 1936 Midwives' Act made all LSAs responsible for providing an adequate salaried domiciliary midwifery service. In Scotland, the Maternity Services Act of 1937 also entitled all pregnant women to the services of a doctor if they gave birth at home (Towler & Bramall, 1986) Under the 1936 Midwives' Act, midwives had to attend a 7-day refresher course every 5 years, to remain eligible to practise, and the title 'Supervisor of Midwives' replaced 'Inspector'. It was considered that this person should be the 'counsellor and friend of the midwives, rather than a relentless critic', and have the 'essential qualities of sympathy and tact' (Ministry of Health 1937).

Having been able to compete with doctors by offering a cheaper service, private midwives could not compete with the subsidised state services. Private midwifery did not fit into the structure of midwifery care in Britain, and by the 1930s independent midwives were a dying breed (Dingwall et al 1988). By 1942, only 2000 out of 15 000 midwives were in private practice (Towler & and Bramall 1986)

Cronk (1990) described how an old midwife advised her to 'get the fees paid before the tears of gratitude are out of their eyes'. This midwife had a great struggle to make ends meet and had to overbook clients to make a living. Although such conditions cannot be in the interests of midwives or mothers. Cronk (1990) felt that midwives made a political mistake in 1948 by becoming salaried employees of the NHS rather than contracted practitioners like GPs. It is easy, however, to understand the lure of regular salaried employment with paid time off. In the NHS women were assured of a doctor if they needed one, and doctors were available at the municipal clinics, but, as Cronk (1990) pointed out, somehow this developed into a presumption that all women must see a doctor.

During the 1930s more registered nurses entered midwifery, because from 1916 they could do a shorter midwifery course than women without a nursing qualification. By 1936, most pupil midwives were registered nurses (Dingwall et al 1988). Wagner (1986) suggested that entry of nurses to midwifery training reduced the power and status of midwives. Nurses are socialized into a medically dominated hierarchy and are focused upon pathology rather than normality. The decline in direct entry midwifery training continued; by 1987 it was offered in only one midwifery school in Britain (Downe 1987). Despite a resurgence in direct entry midwifery courses in the early 1990s, all midwifery courses now tend to be defined around the possession of a nursing qualification (pre- and post-registration courses).

## Subordination of midwifery and fragmentation of care

The subordinate position of the midwife in the new NHS of the early 1950s was reinforced, as the GP was a pregnant woman's first point of contact (Dingwall et al 1988, Robinson 1990). If a doctor and a midwife were present at a delivery together, the doctor had superior status and the midwife was redefined as a maternity nurse (Oakley 1984). As more women gave birth in hospital, more midwives practised in hospital and the absorption of the midwife into the 'maternity nurse' role became complete. Doctors dominated not only the abnormal cases but also determined policies for women having normal pregnancies.

During the 1950s and 1960s, hospitals gave antenatal care to women booked to deliver in them, and most mothers remained in hospital for 10 days so they received all their postnatal care there too (Robinson 1990). There was continuity of care for women whether they chose to deliver at home with their midwife or GP, or in hospital, since the same practitioners provided all the care. As the number of hospital births increased, however, maternity care became fragmented and shared within 'multidisciplinary teams'. DeVries (1989) described the deleterious effect of such teamwork on the relationship between the midwife and the woman. Antenatal care became divided between hospital and community, and maternity units were specialised into departments (antenatal, labour and postnatal). By 1979 64% of midwives were, at any one time, working solely in one speciality (Robinson 1990).

Until 1974, domiciliary midwives had been managed by local government health authorities. The 1973 NHS Reorganisation Act brought domiciliary midwives under the control of hospital midwifery managers, thus integrating all midwifery services within the NHS. Statutory responsibilities for midwives moved from local government health authorities to regional health authorities (or 'Health Boards' in Scotland) of the NHS. Further legislation in 1979 combined the nine bodies concerned with the statutory regulation of nursing, midwifery and health visiting into one body: the United Kingdom Central Council for Nursing, Midwifery and Health Visiting (UKCC). This came about despite the concern of the outgoing Central Midwives' Board that the midwifery profession's independence would be engulfed by the new statutory framework (Towler & Bramall, 1986). The LSA (in practice, the Regional Nursing Officer) now appoints Supervisors of Midwives.

During the 1970s the prevailing medical view was that 'birth is only normal in retrospect' and as Kirkham (1983) asserted: 'by this logic the midwife as a practitioner in her own right is defined out of existence'.

As medical dominance became more blatant, e.g. with routine induction of labour and episiotomy, there was a backlash from consumers and from some midwives. The Association of Radical Midwives (ARM) was formed in 1976, out of concern about the erosion of the midwife's role and the lack of choice for childbearing women (Scruggs et al 1978). Two consumer organisations were active. The National Childbirth Trust (NCT), began to challenge medical authority (Kitzinger 1990) and the Association for Improvements in Maternity Services (AIMS) began to campaign against routine interventions (Tew 1990). During the 1980s, when home births had declined to around 1% in Britain, and many women were denied a home birth by obstructive doctors and midwives, there was growing evidence that birth at home was not necessarily any less safe than in hospital (Campbell & MacFarlane 1987)

## THE PRESENT: THE RISE OF INDEPENDENT MIDWIFERY

During the 1980s, NHS midwives had been attempting to exert more autonomy and improve the system by experimenting with alternative patterns of care (Flint & Poulengeris 1987, Waterhouse 1989). More evidence emerged about good perinatal outcomes for women cared for in low-tech community-based systems (Campbell et al 1991)

With the growth of the alternative childbirth movement,

midwives began to set up in private practice. These self-employed midwives offered, to women who could pay, an option not available to many on the NHS, i.e. delivery at home by a midwife known to them who believes in home birth. As Wagner (1986) stated:

the most effective challenge possible to the male hegemony of the modern, technological medical world, lies in the domain of independent domiciliary practice

Flint (1990) explained why it is important for women to have power over birth in this way. The women constructing this system of care challenge the status quo.

During the mid-1980s approximately 10 midwives practised independently in Britain (Demilew 1991). By 1990, there were 32 independent midwives (Leap 1991) and in 1991 there were 44 (Demilew 1991). By 1994, the estimated number of independent midwives was approximately 100 with 80 belonging to the Independent Midwives Association (Hobbs 1994)[1].

## CLINICAL PRACTICE: THE EXPERIENCE OF INDIVIDUALS

A study (Isherwood 1989a) of independent midwifery was undertaken in 1987–88. This was no more than a pilot study, or initial survey, of independent midwives; there was little information available at that time which was a shortcoming in the knowledge base of the midwifery profession. The time available for the project was 6 months part-time, during which 11 fully established independent midwives and seven occasionally practising independent midwives were included in the study. According to the figures given by Leap (1991) and Demilew (1991) these probably represented most but not all of such practitioners at the time. There were also five formerly independent midwives.

Information was gathered by three methods:

1. questionnaires completed by midwives,
2. tape recorded semi-structured interviews with 21 of the total of 23 midwives, eight clients and four Supervisors of Midwives, and

[1] The Independent Midwives Association, c/o Lesley Hobbs, Nightingale Cottage, Shamblehurst Lane, Botley, Hampshire

3. a diary of observation visits made with six midwives as they practised.

The interviews were conducted in a place of the interviewee's choice. Guidelines were used, but the interviews remained as flexible as possible in terms of length and order of topics, and the interviewee was asked whether she had anything to add on completion of the session. Some interviews were transcribed during the fieldwork, but due to lack of time, many were not transcribed until afterwards. Initially, every word was transcribed, but this proved very time-consuming and it became apparent that only the relevant parts of conversations were needed.

The transcripts were analysed accordance with the 'key' topics in the guidelines and analysis also included any of the spontaneous comments which occurred.

The data presented in this chapter are taken from the study (Isherwood 1989a) unless otherwise stated.

## Reasons for choosing independent practice

Reasons for midwives setting up independently have been given as follows (Isherwood 1989a,b, Demilew 1991):

- Rejection of a medical model of birth.
- Inability to provide satisfactory care in the NHS.
- To maintain the status of midwives as practitioners.
- To give continuity of care and enable women to give birth at home in the manner of their choice.

Independent midwives have made the following comments about choosing independent practice:

... to be a professional in my own right ... what I saw in hospital practice was midwives not working as midwives at all but as obstetric nurses ...

(Demilew 1991)

I wanted to separate myself from a medical view of birth, I felt it was undermining women a lot ...

Women don't have any control ... seeing all the problems and the horrific pain women go through ... I just felt it was so dangerous, women being in hospital ...

## Booking for care

It was found in the study (Isherwood 1989a), that there was usually a 'first point of contact' telephone call from the client, when the midwife explained how she worked and that free homebirth was available on the NHS. The fee was often discussed and the client would either spend some time thinking about it or would arrange a booking visit. Criteria for booking were not always in accordance with conventional medical and midwifery risk factors:

We haven't refused anybody. I feel women select themselves. I'm certainly not worried by a 'primip' in her thirties. I'm beginning to wonder what *are* the contraindications [to home birth]?

(Isherwood 1989a)

As Leap (1991) has explained, independent midwives did not go out of their way to attract 'abnormal' cases such as breech presentations or twin pregnancies (although Cronk (1990) described how these were considered midwives' cases in her area between 1958 and 1962). Independent midwives remained supportive of women who had decided to give birth at home, with the knowledge of the risks involved, although individual attitudes vary:

IM: I did refuse to take on one woman who lived 30 miles away who had had a previous Caesarean section ... I can't say I'd never book someone with a previous Caesarean but I can't say I'm happy about it.
Q: Primips you're not worried about?
IM: No, I'm not worried about booking older women either. I wouldn't book anybody who had a breech baby ... but we've had quite a few ... who have had a previous postpartum haemorrhage and one with a retained placenta. With that sort of thing, I always look at the reasons ...

Q: What about obstetric or medical condition ... do you ever find something at booking that gives you second thoughts?
IM: Yes, but I don't drop them! I still book them ....

*(Isherwood 1989a)*

## Antenatal care

When an independent midwife books a woman for delivery at home, she informs the local Supervisor of Midwives. This may involve notifying her Intention to Practice (a form which has to be completed annually by all practising midwives, and when a midwife intends to practise in an LSA area where she has not done so before). She obtains the necessary forms from the

Supervisor of Midwives and clarifies the arrangements for supervision and emergency services.

The study (Isherwood 1989a) found that blood tests were either arranged through the GP if there was one covering or by the midwife herself. In the latter case, the blood could be tested privately and the costs passed on to the client, but if there was a good relationship with the Supervisor of Midwives, the Supervisor might arrange for the testing to be done through the NHS. Ultrasound and other tests, if necessary, were similarly obtained. Independent midwives were generally willing to liaise with GPs for obstetric cover, whilst not allowing the absence of a GP to worry them unduly.

Antenatal care usually took place in the midwife's or the client's home. When midwives were working in a partnership, antenatal care was usually shared, so that both midwives met the client.

## Intrapartum care

When a client went into labour, she contacted her midwife, or, in a partnership, the midwife on call. It was found that independent midwives usually carry radio pagers and many also used telephone answering machines. Labour and birth took place at home unless complications arose requiring hospital transfer.

Few of the midwives carried analgesics such as pethidine, but many had Entonox machines (to provide nitrous oxide gas). They had supplies of emergency drugs (e.g. syntometrine, ergometrine and oxygen) and equipment; several midwives also had intubation and intravenous equipment.

Some midwives and clients used alternative therapies. A natural birth was the aim of client and midwife; active positions were favoured for the birth. Independent midwives talked about 'catching' babies rather than delivering them (Isherwood 1989a).

If a woman needed transfer to hospital this might be arranged directly, by the midwife via the Supervisor of Midwives, or via the GP. Obstetric referral rates for three midwives are shown in Table 2.1.

## Postnatal care

If a client delivered in hospital, the midwife usually visited her there until she went home. Otherwise postnatal care took place, as

**Table 2.1** Independent midwife referral rates (based on the total number of births reported) (Isherwood 1989a)

|                       | Midwife 1 | Midwife 2 | Midwife 3 |
|-----------------------|-----------|-----------|-----------|
| Total births          | 109       | 90        | 61        |
| Home births           | 84        | 70        | 54        |
| Antenatal transfers   | 4         | 11        | 0*        |
| Intrapartum transfers | 21        | 9         | 5         |
| Postnatal transfers   | 2         | 0         | 1         |

* Two women had planned hospital deliveries

usual, in the mother's home up to the 28th day. However, many midwives maintained a social relationship with their clients well beyond this time. There was a great deal of support between independent midwives and their clients (Isherwood 1989a)

## Workload

The average number of births attended by fully established independent midwives was 2.2 per month (Isherwood 1989a). The work, however, was erratic; there were no births in some months and in others as many as four or five. Although the numbers of clients were not very great, the midwives spent much time on call.

Other aspects of the workload were dependent upon the relationship with the Supervisor of Midwives. If it was not good, a midwife had to spend much time solving a basic problem, such as obtaining access to blood test, etc.

In many cases, a midwife had to liaise with people who did not know what an independent midwife was. Some midwives had to accept clients who lived far away, as they were financially dependent on clients who could afford to pay a fee.

## REASONS FOR BOOKING WITH AN INDEPENDENT MIDWIFE

The main reasons (Isherwood 1989a) given by clients and midwives for booking an independent midwife were:

• Wanting to know the person who was going to deliver their baby and having trust in them.

- Wishing to give birth at home (not always a primary reason for booking with an independent midwife).
- Wishing to have as little intervention as possible during pregnancy and labour
- Rejection of the NHS, based on prior obstetric experience or NHS care during pregnancy

## Home birth and safety

The place of birth was not important to all women. Some clients did not want a home birth initially but wanted a midwife they knew and trusted. By talking with the midwife, the pros and cons were clarified. Many midwives felt that the swing to encouraging 100% birth in hospital was not necessarily safer for all women:

> IM: Being in hospital isn't a total safeguard . . . I'm not going to say that home is the safest place for every woman. Of course it isn't, but I think the majority of woman should have the option of home birth if they want it. One of the main reasons for working independently is that I feel home is a far safer place.
> Q: Do you think that women are allowed to make an informed choice about having a baby in hospital?
> IM: Oh, no . . .

Another midwife discussed the issue of power:

> They know they can't have me unless it's a home birth . . . We talk a lot about . . . going into hospital . . . and the penny kind of drops about who has got control and who has got the power. Women don't want to give up that stuff, you know. And that's universal. I found that out as an NCT teacher . . . I'll never forget the look on the faces of the labour ward staff when a very young black woman asserted herself and said 'What's that for? Do I have to have it?'

An experienced midwife made the following comment:

> The safety of birth is not about the machines in the place, and the beds that go up and down . . . and how many doctors . . . it's about a skilled practitioner who is intelligent about what she does, and who knows the limit of safety and of practice, and respects those. And who respects the normal birth process, and is willing to be flexible and go with it, even if it's sometimes outside her experience, initially . . . but to be open to that. That's what makes it safe.

With women for whom birth at home was important, independent midwives said they made it clear that a home birth with an NHS midwife was free. Several clients had been told that they might have one of several NHS midwives; up to 24 in one case (Isherwood 1989a). This was unacceptable to these women.

## Experiences of clients

Cecile, a 31-year-old black woman, was very unhappy with her first birth experience in a London hospital:

It was one o'clock in the morning and . . . I was having strong contractions but not dilating at all. They had wired me up to the monitor, with the electrode . . . they turned to my partner and said 'She's not going to deliver until morning, go home and sleep'. I had pethidine . . . couldn't remember my breathing . . . it was panic and nobody was with me. By the time the day staff came on, I was well advanced and said I felt like pushing . . . loads of people appeared and I had a junior student . . . deliver, Not even a midwife . . . a doctor . . . I had my legs in stirrups. My partner got there too late. They did a routine episiotomy . . . I felt I had no control over the birth. I was most put out that this strange young man had done the delivery, and rather brutally. To have my legs in stirrups was the most humiliating and degrading experience.

When Cecile became pregnant again, she decided to book with an independent midwife already known to her:

The more I found out about home birth, the more I felt it would be nice, but I would be scared of what could go wrong. But I made the decision that I would like to have a home birth and certainly want (an independent midwife) and her partner to deliver my baby. I knew them as friends, I trusted them . . . that was important . . . and unique to have somebody you know and care about to deliver your baby, as opposed to those faceless medics.

Hannah was a 40-year-old white woman. She had not been happy with her first birth experience in hospital and the baby died from birth asphyxia. Her next baby was born in hospital and the experience was unpleasant:

I hadn't considered a home birth after . . . the first time, but I did hate the time in hospital . . . When I was pregnant with my third baby, the community midwives accepted me for the 'DOMINO' scheme. But the registrar warned me that I would be monitored from 1 cm dilation, despite my requesting an active birth . . . I came away feeling that I didn't ever want to go near them again . . . I wanted to get it right, to have it the way I wanted . . .'

Hannah decided to have her baby at home with an independent midwife:

We were very impressed with how thorough she was (the midwife) without being intrusive . . . I felt very strongly that it must be a very private thing. She also knew me, knew what I wanted, and treated me with respect, which I don't feel I have ever received from the medical

profession ... I didn't like the community midwives I had met. They
didn't seem interested ... it was just a job to them. I think it should
be possible on the NHS, for everyone who wants it, to have
somebody looking after you throughout pregnancy ... I know I'm
privileged ... I can pay, but it is a good model for care.

(Isherwood 1989a)

## FURTHER ASPECTS OF INDEPENDENT MIDWIFERY

### Transfer to hospital

Women who were transferred to hospital suffered great disappointment, but accepted that it had been necessary:

Q:  When someone has needed to be transferred, are their feelings towards you any
different?
IM: Their feelings, on the whole, tend to be that it didn't really matter. They could
handle it because they were surrounded with such total love and support. And
when you've got that, and are treated with respect, anything is OK. There is
disappointment, but they know they did everything possible to have it the way
they wanted. They weren't forced into anything.

### Private practice

Independent midwives are 'private' midwives because they
charge a fee for their services. However, they accept lower fees or
payment in kind in the case of financial difficulty for the client
(Isherwood 1989a, Leap 1991). The motive underlying the midwives' practice seems not to be that of profit, but of giving a
service where it is needed while making enough to live on. The
fees are relatively low (Table 2.2). They seem to be a compromise

**Table 2.2**  Fees for full independent midwifery
care (1987–1988) (Isherwood 1989a)

|  | £ |
| --- | --- |
| London | 700–800 |
| Scotland | 600 |
| Brighton | 500–600 |
| Worcestershire | 500 |
| Merseyside | 450 |
| Humberside | 400 |
| Manchester/Lancashire | 200–400 |
| Lincolnshire | 100–200 |

between what the midwife deserves, what she can live on and what a client may reasonably be expected to pay:

Hannah: It was worth every penny of the £700. I costed out the midwife's time and it came to about £10 per hour.

Q: Do your clients ever moan about how much you charge?
IM: People are quite shocked at how much it is, sometimes; other people think it's quite cheap . . . People underrate how much time and commitment goes into it, from the midwife.
Q: Do you charge as much if someone else has to deliver them in hospital?'
IM: Yes . . . I sometimes think I ought to charge them double if they are transferred! It takes years off my life . . .!

Attitudes to private practice varied between midwives. Some detested having to charge and wanted their type of service to be available on the NHS; others felt that they could never work in the same way within the NHS.

Q: How do you feel about charging . . . and private practice?
IM: I am very happy . . . My only qualm is that I do feel it should be on the NHS. I need to live but I think the NHS should pay me, not the women.
IM: I suppose, ideologically, I like the idea of the NHS. Practically . . . it's not working in terms of providing good care or a satisfying place for people to work. Anything really progressive, you're not going to get in the NHS. So do you forgo it or look elsewhere?

Some midwives felt it was important for a client to show that she valued the midwife by paying a fee and they had no reservations about charging. As the above discussion demonstrated, independent midwifery points to a need which is not met by the maternity services in some places. One independent midwife rarely practised in one local area:

I work mainly in X Health Authority . . . not so much in Y because they have wonderful community midwives. Where there's a good home birth service . . . I don't practise. I refer the women to the community midwives because they should get the service free.

## Indemnity insurance

Many midwives practise in pairs or flexible groups (Isherwood 1989a, Demilew 1991, Leap 1991). Unlike midwives in the NHS, they supply their own equipment and pay for their statutory refresher courses. Until the end of 1993, membership of the Royal College of Midwives (RCM) provided indemnity insurance up to £2 million. However, following two claims brought against independent midwives, the insurance company serving the RCM increased the premium required for these practitioners to well above the premium for those practising within the NHS.

At the time of writing, a difficult choice was faced by the RCM. Independent midwives might be excluded from RCM membership on the grounds of cost; or the vastly increased premium could be paid, leading to cuts in staff and services to members, or all 36 000 members could be balloted about their willingness to pay an extra £16 to cover the additional premium needed by independent midwives.

The implications for independent practice are immense. Most independent midwives will never earn sufficient sums to pay an individual indemnity premium which might be as high as £3000. If they are compelled to cease practising (ironically, by the free market forces in the insurance industry) then choice of childbearing women will be more limited. The stimulus of independent midwifery will no longer be there to influence the new and evolving NHS systems which may arise from the reports of the committees chaired by Winterton and Cumberledge (Select Committee on Health 1992, Department of Health 1993). It remains to be seen whether the insurance market succeeds in splitting the midwifery profession or whether NHS midwives unite to support their independent colleagues.

## Accountability

Two of the reasons for practising independently are related to the role of the midwife. Independent midwives have mostly worked within the NHS and then have left, feeling unable to work within the constraints they encountered there, although Demilew (1991) reported a recent increase in midwives setting up independently with no prior practice as an NHS midwife. Another reason given was to keep alive the principle that midwives was empowered by law to practise independently:

Q: Why do you feel independent midwifery is important for midwifery?
IM: Because of the principle that midwives can work in that way . . . that we don't have to consult the local doctor.
Q: What do you say . . . to student midwives about being an independent practitioner . . . are you different from any other midwife?
IM: No! That's the big message I have for them! They often say: do you have special insurance? And I say: well, do you? I'm as accountable for my practice as you are. Just because you are part of a hierarchy and have got a red panic button to press, it doesn't mean you are less accountable . . . midwives in the NHS are

as accountable as I am. They may not feel it, because of that sense of there always being someone above them.

Some independent midwives feel that most midwives do not really want a great deal of responsibility:

Midwives . . . want to have their cake and eat it. To have the glory of being practitioners, but when it actually comes to standing up for what you believe in, that's a very different story . . . there has to be a real willingness to commit (yourself). I just don't feel this is the case for midwives as a group of women. And there is a lot of fear. Midwives are full of fear of birth.

Independent midwives believed that working outside the NHS helped them to fulfil the role of the midwife better:

You can formulate your own policies . . . Most NHS midwives are overworked . . . I have more time to analyse and think about the care I give. Working with another independent midwife, we bounce ideas off each other . . . I think midwives need more freedom to find out things. We don't learn from obstetrics, we've got to learn from ourselves.

## The Supervisor of Midwives

Independent midwives had various reactions to supervision:

I think independent midwifery is good for the whole system of supervision of midwives. It is probably the first time the supervisor has had to separate her role of manager and supervisor, because she can't manage us, she can't suspend us from duty . . . it's purely midwifery supervision and she has to support us in what we do. I think the role of the supervisor is a very good thing.

I've never had any real problems with supervisors. I've never expected to . . . I've always approached them as if they are there to support me . . . consulted with them . . . asked them for advice and support, and put it in those terms.

IM: Most are uninterfering . . . try to be helpful. Some . . . how the hell they got into that position, God only knows. I don't.
Q:  Do you think supervisors receive adequate preparation?
IM: No, I've had so many different things said about what has to be done.
Q:  Do you think they ever confuse the roles of supervisor and manager?
IM: Some . . . are clear. Most . . . get it muddled initially.

Independent midwifery makes the role of Supervisor of Midwives clear. Supervisory responsibilities have not altered greatly, despite changes in the maternity services and conditions in which midwives practise. Supervision is usually left to midwifery managers, whose responsibilities may clash (Isherwood 1988). Demilew (1991) suggested that the midwifery profession has attempted to control independent midwives by strict supervision with an unduly high rate of disciplinary action. Independent midwives felt supervision was exercised in a controlling way, obstructing clients from getting quality care.

Demilew (1991) suggests that tension between independent and NHS midwives exists because of different ideas about birth; about what being a practitioner means; what supervision is for, and how it should be practised. She reported that one-third of the independent midwives felt there was no place for midwifery supervision.

## THE FUTURE?

The word 'independent' has very special and important connotations for British midwives, who see the emphasis more on autonomy of practice than on employment status. Despite not always being accepted or even welcomed by some members of their own profession, independent midwives still practise; sometimes under difficult circumstances and sometimes without professional support. They do so to provide what they believe to be good and appropriate care for women and to fulfil the true role of the midwife.

Demilew (1991) suggests that independent midwives are redefining the meaning of 'professional', i.e. they have equal but complementary responsibility within a relationship of trust and mutual respect with the client, rather than exerting professional authority from a distance.

The present system whereby most women book under consultant care is not appropriate for the majority of women who have a normal pregnancy and labour. But for more appropriate maternity care and for midwives' skills to be used fully, there would also have to be:

- midwives able to work as independent practitioners in a system which supports them as clinicians,
- greater awareness of the role of the midwife amongst the general public, the midwifery and medical professions, and
- fundamental changes in the way women book for maternity care and in where maternity care is based.

## CONCLUSION

The basis upon which midwives are employed in the NHS does not reflect their status in law as independent practitioners. By contracting into the NHS, midwives could achieve professional autonomy similar to that of GPs and dentists. The NHS in Britain is undergoing massive changes, and market forces are to be allowed into health care provision. It remains to be seen for how long maternity care will remain available for 'free' on the NHS. Pregnancy is, after all, a largely avoidable and voluntary condition. But should childbearing women have to pay to receive optimal care? Midwifery, in its true sense, has been shown to be a cost-effective way of delivery maternity care and should therefore be attractive to the policy makers. Independent midwifery may serve to remind all midwives of what it means to be a midwife, and provide us with an ideal model of care.

REFERENCES

Campbell R, Macfarlane A 1987 Where to be born? The debate and the evidence National Perinatal Epidemiology Unit, Oxford
Campbell R, Macfarlane A, Cavenagh S 1991 Choice and chance in low-risk maternity care. British Medical Journal 303: 1487–1488
Cronk M 1990 Midwifery: a practitioner's view from within the National Health Service. Midwife, Health Visitor and Community Nurse 26(3): 58–63
Demilew J 1991 The struggle to practise: a sociological analysis of the crisis within the British midwifery profession. Unpublished MSc dissertation, South Bank Polytechnic, London
Department of Health 1993 Changing childbirth Part 1. Report of the Expert Maternity Group (Chair Cumberledge J). HMSO, London
DeVries R 1989 Caregivers in pregnancy and childbirth. In: Enkin M, Chalmers I, Keirse M (eds) Effective care in pregnancy and childbirth. Oxford University Press, Oxford
Dingwall R, Rafferty A, Webster C 1988 An introduction to the social history of nursing. Routledge London
Donnison J 1977 Midwives and medical men: a history of the struggle for the control of childbirth. Heinmann, London
Downe S 1987 Direct entry training – the future for English midwifery? Proceedings of the 21st International Confederation of Midwives Conference August 24th, The Hague, Netherlands, p 21–24
Flint C 1990 Power over birth – its importance for women. Obstetric and Gynaecology Product News, Spring: 16–17
Flint C, Poulengeris P 1987 Know your midwife. Private publication
Hobbs L 1994 Personal communication
Isherwood K 1988 Friend or watchdog? Nursing Times 84(24): 65
Isherwood K 1989a, Independent midwifery in the United Kingdom 1987–1988. Unpublished study supported by the Royal College of Midwives Trust and

Farley's Health Product Award for Midwives, 1987

Isherwood K 1989b, Independent midwifery in the UK Midwife, Health Visitor and Community Nurse 25(7): 307–309

Kirkham M J 1983, Labouring in the dark: limitation of the giving of information to enable patients to orientate themselves to the likely events and time scale of labour. In: Wilson-Barnett J (ed) Nursing research: ten studies of patient care John Wiley, Chichester, Sussex

Kitzinger J 1990 Strategies of the early childbirth movement: a case study of the National Childbirth Trust. In: Garcia J, Kilpatrick R, Richards M (eds) The politics of maternity care: services for childbearing women in twentieth-century Britain. Croom Helm, London

Leap N 1991, Independent midwifery – filling the gaps and picking up the pieces, Midwives Chronicle 104(1237): 34–38

Ministry of Health 1937, Supervision of midwives. Circular 1620, May 7. HMSO, London

Oakley A 1984 The captured womb: a history of the medical care of pregnant women. Blackwell, Oxford

Robinson S 1990 Maintaining the independence of the midwifery profession: a continuing struggle. In: Garcia J, Kilpatrick R, Richards M (eds) The politics of maternity care: services for childbearing women in twentieth-century Britain. Croom Helm, London

Scruggs M, Rose S, Jury L 1978 On her own responsibility Association of Radical Midwives Newsletter (1) June, p 4–5

Select Committee on Health 1992 Maternity services: second report of the House of Commons Health Committee (Chair Winterton N). HMSO, London

Tew M 1990 Safer childbirth? a critical history of maternity care. Chapman and Hall, London

Towler J, Bramall J 1986 Midwives in history and society. Croom Helm, London

Wagner M 1986, The medicalisation of birth In: Claxton R (ed) Birth matters: issues and alternatives in childbirth. Unwin Paperbacks, London.

Waterhouse I 1989 Oh to be a midwife: the Reading model. Midwife Health Visitor and Community Nurse 29(9): 395–396

# 3

# Independent midwifery in Australia

*Maggie Lecky-Thompson*

## INTRODUCTION

Independent midwifery in Australia was at a critical point in the early 1990s, struggling for survival at a time of great change. Three factors worked against midwifery: medical dominance, antagonism by the nursing profession and ignorance within the community about the role of a midwife. The medical dominance had been brought about in part by the training of more doctors per head of population than was necessary (Willis 1989)

This is a feature in midwives' struggles in other countries (Chs 4 and 7 by Donley and Roberts). The nursing profession in Australia denies the right of midwives to a separate professional identity. With this powerful alliance in force, the fewer and less militant midwives are constantly overruled. Australian women are largely unaware of the role of the midwife and that, with midwives whose status was high, they could be supported to regain their rights and power in childbirth.

There are approximately 70 000 trained midwives, however only 10 000 are practising. The New South Wales (NSW) Department of Health figures suggest that only 25% of those registered are actually working as midwives. There are approximately 200 000 births annually in Australia and of these about 1000 babies are born at home with care from about 100 independent midwives. A handful of these midwives are unregistered.

These independent midwives used as role model midwives from our own past, together with some present day midwives of Europe and the Americas. It is from the work of these independent midwives, and their supporting clientele, that the impetus for change and improvement in maternity care is developing.

Independent midwifery in Australia grew out of a demand from women who wanted to have options, and to avoid the common experience in the 1960s and 1970s, that is, the disempowerment of a hospital birth. Some midwives were equally dissatisfied with their diminishing role within hospitals and in other Government-funded community positions.

Greater options in midwifery services are evolving and emerging at a time when fewer medical graduates are choosing the long preparation to become obstetricians. This is due in part to medical insurance premiums, which are becoming exorbitant at a time when it is feared that Australia will follow the American path of more and greater litigation. These influences clearly alter individual practices with a consequent tussle for power between obstetricians and midwives.

The adversaries are not simply the providers of maternity care; their differing and at times opposing philosophies and models of care are also jostling for supremacy. The debate is seen by many as a feminist issue, men versus women. This is at its strongest among the aboriginal community where birthing has always been 'women's business'.

## POLITICAL BACKGROUND

At the last two federal elections it was clear that both major political parties were in favour of midwives giving maternity care rather than doctors because of politicians' awareness of the enormous cost savings to be obtained.

The Labour Federal Government under Hawke had launched a remodelled social health package in 1983, called Medicare. A similar package had been introduced in the 1970s under Whitlam, the Labour leader of the day. Medicare made 'free' health care possible, but it was only free in a limited sense as there was a 2% tax levy on wage earners.

In late 1993 and early 1994 the Western Australia Minister for

Health, Peter Foss lobbied the Federal Government for a Medicare rebate for families choosing a home birth. His interest and commitment sprang from the births of three of his four children having taken place at home, with independent midwife care. The Conservative Medical Associations were incensed by his position and at the time of writing (March 1994), are making his portfolio very difficult.

## Reviews of maternity care

Throughout the 1980s and early 1990s all of the eight state and territory governments, with the exception of Queensland, reviewed their maternity care. The reports varied in their titles, from 'obstetrical' to 'maternity' to 'birthing' reviews, but had similar structures and recommendations. Apart from in the Northern Territory and Australian Capital Territory, all the reviews were chaired either by obstetricians or epidemiologists. South Australia, Western Australia, Victoria and NSW established task forces which called for written submissions, and also set up meetings at public places to invite comments from the general population. The submissions were allocated to a variety of working parties.

Unlike the recent British reviews chaired by Winterton and Cumberledge (Committee on Select Health 1992, Department of Health 1993) their Australian counterparts were delegated by the politicians to obstetricians, with approximately half the chairs taken by women. There were only a token number of consumers, and in the majority of cases the latter were unable to contribute to a clear community focus, due to the dominance held by the stakeholders. Nonetheless, many remarkable and innovative recommendations were made that set out a path for more birth options, and some that would give restricted rights of practice to midwives. In fact, getting these recommendations implemented has been exceedingly difficult in many area health services.

In early 1994 the National Health and Medical Research Council (NHMRC) circulated a draft document *Effective Care in Childbirth* (NHMRC 1994) . This is a preparatory step for issuing regulatory recommendations about childbirth in Australia. Submissions have been sought about this most recent national statement, which is intended to update all the state reviews. Consumer membership consisted of two women from the Consumers' Health Forum, a bureau within the NHMRC which does not necessarily have any ties with grassroots consumer groups. In addition, there were two midwives from South Australia and one from NSW.

There were 15 recommendations in the draft document and many reflect great progress for midwifery. It is clear, however, that some motivating factors have been the reality of soaring medical indemnity costs, and the fact that obstetricians need to acknowledge the responsibility that GPs and midwives assume in the more rural and remote areas.

The recommendations included some that have already been implemented in most states for the past 5 years, such as visiting rights for independent midwives, limited prescribing rights and the lifting of restrictions on the power of midwives to order a range of tests for the care of 'normal pregnancy in a healthy woman'. There was a recommendation to support the funding of care for 'the woman and her baby in a domiciliary setting'. This, however, was not support for home birth but for early discharge from hospital. The report was disappointing in that it did not take the leap of recognising the benefits of continuity of care, whether as continuity of a single carer or from a small team of midwives. When the word 'team' was mentioned, it was in the context of a collaborative approach of all stakeholders. There was a call for funding for evaluation and research into new initiatives, but this was apparently addressed to the private sector as there was no commitment from the federal treasury. The recommendation to support a national register of midwives was welcomed.

## Birth centres in Australia

Birth centres in Australia opened in the late 1970s. Many midwife managers were inspired by American birth centres, and set about establishing free-standing, midwife-staffed facilities with the options of baths, rooms to accommodate families and children-friendly environments. This idea quickly became diluted so that the only free-standing birth centre in Australia is a private building in Victoria, owned and operated by an obstetrician supported by a team of midwives. There are varying degrees of obstetrician and GP involvement between the different units.

Not all states have birth centres. Victoria has always had the most (approximately eight), and under the patronage of the doctors who run them, they have proved to be a success. Western

Australia is due to open its first at the King Edward Memorial Hospital. This hospital did open a birth centre 10 years ago, but it was closed as the general opinion was that it was not necessary because the labour ward was so good. The Northern Territory does not have any birth centres, and the first in Queensland opens in 1994. There is one birth centre in the Australian Capital Territory, which the obstetricians refuse to attend, thus allowing GPs and midwives to work unimpeded.

Sydney, Australia's biggest city, has a handful of birth centres and there are a few more in the country areas of New South Wales, a total of nine in the State. None are free-standing. The Launceston birth centre is unique. Established in the early 1980s, it is the property of that State's branch of the Childbirth Education Association. It was the first, and still is the only birth centre to be owned by a consumer group who employ the midwives. In some instances these midwives are traditional midwives, and they have earned great respect in the community.

## HEALTH AND NURSES' ACTS

Each of the eight states and territories has different legislation governing the role and practice of midwifery. These are the Health Acts and the Nurses' Acts.

There is no longer provision for a separate midwifery register in any of the states: all midwives come under the broad category of 'nurse'. Since the 1950s, midwives in Victoria have been severely limited in their independent role by legislation which prohibits a woman from seeking care from anyone other than a doctor during her pregnancy. In Tasmania, it is the midwives who must be 'legally responsible' to the registered medical practitioner. In both States, if a midwife gives advice to a pregnant women, this can be considered 'care', and in certain circumstances the midwife is liable to be deregistered.

Unfortunately, in Victoria and in the Australian Capital Territory, several doctors who have given support to midwives in the past for home births, have now been warned by their medical defence union to desist from this. It is seen that doctors alone would take the brunt of medical litigation. In the late 1980s and early 1990s in Victoria, there were a number of instances of doctors being sued. Whenever this happens, there is adverse publicity about home births, despite the fact that none of the recent court cases have been concerned with home births. Midwives insist that they are professionally responsible, and capable of making their own clinical judgements. These principles, however, are rejected: on the one hand by doctors who do not wish to acknowledge midwives' competencies, and on the other hand by more conservative groups of nurses and midwives, who fear the changes greater autonomy and responsibility could make for them. It would not be surprising if midwifery care was once again driven underground by a fear of litigation. This would, of course, hamper the choices available to women.

During the 1970s, the State of Victoria had the largest proportion of home births, for its population, of any state. There was a large number of lay midwives who were not as limited as the registered midwives. Bob Hawke's first grandchild was born at home within a month of his election to office as Prime Minister in 1982. The medical fraternity saw this as a possibly fashionable trend which could sweep the nation, and were quick to mount a devastating campaign against a general practitioner in Victoria who undertook a large number of home births. Despite the fact that this GP was not involved in the birth of the Prime Minister's grandchild, and had excellent outcomes of over 1300 home births, the campaign resulted in his deregistration.

In 1982 a much respected Tasmanian midwife was deregistered for 12 months. This deregistration was a result of a home birth. The woman expecting the baby had planned a home birth with the midwife providing care. Even though the baby died prior to birth commencing, the woman still wanted the baby to be born at home and the midwife agreed to help. The midwife was then subject to a Nurses' Registration Board hearing, during which the testimony of the woman played no part and which resulted in the deregistration.

With the exception of Victoria and Tasmania, Australian midwives were permitted to practise in any setting and without the supervision of medical practitioners. Draconian changes in the NSW Nurses' Act 1991 both criminalised traditional midwives, and at the same time authorised nurses to conduct midwifery in hospital settings. In real terms this has meant that area health services need not have the expense of employing more highly qualified staff as long as there is a midwife available at the end of a telephone.

Whereas the vast majority of midwives are registered, and fail to comprehend the feminist and historical repercussions of jailing unqualified women who assist in childbirth, as provided for in the first part of the changed Act, there is a growing awareness, by midwives themselves, about the long-term effects of denigrating the profession by dismissing the importance of a midwife's training and education, which the second change to the Act heralds. It is to be hoped that these midwives will be able to use the governmental political structures to have this law altered.

Northern Territory is poised to embrace the same Act and there is a national movement to standardise all nurses' registration. Midwives do not have a separate registration, however, and they are the only class of 'nurse' who require an 'Authority to Practise'. There are many who see this as pandering to a vocal minority and will work to see the difference between nurses and midwives eradicated.

Traditional midwives, who include aboriginal women in largely rural areas, often live in remote settings. They have a strong pioneering spirit, and have acquired a wide range of skills and knowledge which are not currently available in institutional settings. There is a movement among feminist lawyers to revoke that part of the Act which could have these midwives imprisoned. Clearly the more conservative midwives will seek other routes.

# PROFESSIONAL ORGANISATIONS FOR MIDWIVES

## The Australian College of Midwives Incorporated

The Australian College of Midwives Incorporated (ACMI) was the dream and creation of two midwives from Melbourne and Sydney. Margaret Peters (an administrator from Victoria) and Pamela Hayes (an educator from Sydney) had attended a number of the conferences of the International Confederation of Midwives (ICM), and saw the need and potential for an Australian national college. It began as the National Association of Midwives and had an inaugural conference in 1979. By 1986, the association had achieved the status of college.

The structure allows for each state and territory to have an executive committee. From each of these committees, one national delegate and an alternative are elected and these midwives form the National Executive. The membership of the College has grown, especially in NSW, the state with the largest population.

This growth in membership was boosted by the very successful ICM conference which was held in Sydney in 1983.

The College fulfils a much needed role as the professional voice for midwives. It is representative of the population of midwives, as most the members are employed in hospital. In contrast to the New Zealand College of Midwives (see Ch. 4) whose inaugural members and strengths were drawn from domiciliary midwives, the ACMI has its roots and controlling faction in the educational and administrative sphere. The New Zealand College has always been committed to the consumer's needs and has a strong feminist philosophy, whereas the Australian College is committed to achieving recognition on a professional footing, for example, seeking equality with, and approval from, the medical profession.

The ACMI has enormous problems in being heard alongside the nursing College and unions. These bodies have greater numbers and have been established longer, and therefore have the political advantage. Historically, educationally and in professional groups, midwives in Australia sprang from a nursing base. Early loyalties and ties to nursing have obscured the message that midwifery is best kept well away from the nursing model, a message which does not suit the generalist nursing philosophy which the health departments would rather keep in place.

Some more enlightened obstetricians have welcomed the College and its endeavours. Despite this support, they still try to control and direct the education and practice of midwives. The obstetricians have also arranged restrictions on general practitioners who give maternity care, so midwives are not alone in this.

The NHMRC established three working parties between 1987 and 1991 to examine birth centres and home births, and make recommendations and set guidelines for them. In 1987 the working party recommended that the ACMI be asked to set up an accreditation process for independently practising midwives. The various health department reviews of the maternity services echoed this need. After much deliberation, and some conflict between the independent and hospital-aligned members, the College granted accreditation to some 50–75 midwives. It was agreed that, as this was a new process, adaptation and alteration might be required periodically.

To gain accreditation with the College, a midwife had to demonstrate her capabilities in neonatal resuscitation, in suturing the perineum, and that she had taken responsibility for management throughout labour for at least 10 cases. Evidence of ongoing education and references was also required. Review of the individual accreditation had to take place every 3 years.

Further conflict occurred as the submissions from independent midwives, regarding adaptation and alteration, were ignored. Of the 70 midwives who originally gained accreditation, only four were accepted for reaccreditation. It seems that rather than the empowering, protective and expansive ideology that was evident at the start of this register, there is now an inflexible and bureaucratic programme, emphasising control and restriction rather than expansion and flexibility.

The College has produced standards of practice and from time to time takes as its own policies some of those embraced by the ICM. In early 1994 there was considerable confusion and conflict evident in both state branches and the National Executive.

## The Australian Society of Independent Midwives

Despite the formation of the ACMI, there was a need to represent the voice and situation of the independent midwife, and to support the fact that wherever midwives worked, their right to autonomous practice required recognition. In August 1989 the Australian Society of Independent Midwives (ASIM) was set up. The examples of the Association of Radical Midwives (ARM) in the UK and the Midwives' Alliance of North America (MANA) served as role models, which it was felt were sorely required in Australia.

During the late 1980s there was an urgent need to develop structures to consider the issues of accountability, mediation and conciliation. It was at a time when a number of circumstances came together:

- The federal Government had allocated A$6.4 million to develop alternative birthing services.
- Midwifery education was becoming more like obstetrical nurse training.
- The consumer groups were beginning to disintegrate because the setting up of a number of birth centres had led them to believe that consumer pressure had done its job.
- The ACMI was regarded as the only voice for all midwives, despite the fact that traditionally trained midwives were not only excluded from the College but were victimised by its policies.

There were divisions of opinion in Sydney, and the independent midwives, a small group, had an obvious need of communication with their counterparts in other Australian states. The cost of communication is always a problem in Australia, with the danger of any group becoming insular due to the vast distances. Given the scarcity of independent midwives there was an awareness of how much they needed to know the situation in other states and to develop solidarity.

Following the establishment of the ASIM, representatives from each state were sought who would provide information for a national representative. The national representative acts as the distribution point for the various midwives in their different states. A newsletter, the *Independently Practising Midwives' Communiqué*, had started in October 1988 and eventually this became the *Australian Society of Independent Midwives Communiqué*, edited and published by the ASIM National Representative, Maggie Lecky-Thompson.

The ASIM acts both as a lobby group and an information resource. State representatives were initially shy in coming forward, but more recently area representatives have asked to assist. Whereas Australia is divided into obvious states, there are smaller less distinct 'areas', such as the South Coast, Central Coast and Hunter Areas in NSW, or the Far North in Queensland. Meetings have only been possible at the Homebirth Australia national conferences. The society welcomes a non-elitist policy and equal input from all who support the concepts of independent midwifery. This open structure is challenging to some and welcomed by others.

ASIM has a daunting task ahead. Some state and area branches have been coerced into dropping the title and role of 'independent' from their group names and activities. Two examples of how this can happen are illustrated here.

There is a midwifery group practice in Newcastle, NSW. The members have been pioneers in achieving visiting rights to a major city hospital, where they give total care to women referred to them by obstetricians. They have also set up a 'Know Your Midwife' scheme, and will publish the results of the first 2years of operation in 1994 (Rowley 1994). These midwives have excellent outcomes, especially with high risk women. The doctors referring the women have acknowledged, by continued referral, the benefits of their one-to-one care giving.

In Victoria, midwives were gradually regaining their role, but legislation, which would have recognised the midwives' right to autonomous practice, was withdrawn from Parliament at the eleventh hour as a result of a letter from a female obstetrician which suggested midwives were not sufficiently competent. There is a small but vigorous handful of midwives who choose to give continuity of care at home whenever possible. Both these groups, in Newcastle and Victoria, have been restricted by the fact that obstetricians resent the midwives working independently of their supervision or of that of an institution.

The consequences were that the Newcastle midwives could not attend home births, and the midwives in Victoria have had to remove the word 'Independent' from their title so that 'Midwives in Independent Practice' has now become 'Midwives in Private Practice'.

Maintaining the independence of midwives remains a struggle. There are other factors which help to keep the issues of home births hidden. The collection of data about home births is no longer undertaken nationally, and the recession has driven many women who would like, but cannot afford, home births back to the Medicare-funded hospital systems.

These hospitals still fail to deliver adequate full maternity care. There is a growing expectation that women will leave hospital 24 hours after the birth to go home or book into a private hospital for care. Apparently postnatal services are the most expensive and the most easily neglected.

## FUNDING OF BIRTH SERVICES

Medical practitioners and until recently opticians, have been the only health care service providers whose patients can claim a Medicare rebate. Despite early promises by the Government that Medicare rebates would expand to cover many other health care modalities, and that all referrals should not necessarily have to come 'through the portals of doctors', concerted opposition from medical bodies has been successful in ensuring that this does not occur. The Layton Report (Medicare Benefits Review Committee 1986) revealed:

Of the many medical and paramedical issues raised with this committee, the question of Medicare benefits . . . for registered midwives generated the greatest depth of feeling and strongest organized support (25% of the submissions addressed midwifery and parenting).

The issuing of grants was recommended for the evaluation of independent midwifery practices, but the only proposal included was medically and institutionally governed and was not taken any further.

Health, in financial terms, is a state matter. The Federal Government can make recommendations about the way monies are spent, but there is no jurisdiction to enforce these recommendations. An example of this comes from the 1980s, when a Western Australian senator, Jean Jenkins, was able to push through, at Federal level, a Commonwealth funded Alternative Birthing Services grant (known as the ABS). This was $6.4 million to be spent over the next 4 years. A directive was included that the project should be continued if it was successful.

There was a clear provision that the monies were to go to non-institutional birthing options.

However in NSW the money was divided between aboriginal women's health (all Koori women in NSW deliver in standard hospital wards), and the funding of five full-time midwife positions in birth centres. Although five separate birth centres still receive this funding, not one of them is a free-standing unit. Monies were also distributed in NSW to two Midwives' Teams projects. All the care is delivered within two hospitals.

During the passage of the ABS bill a clause was inserted which required that the midwife involved should not receive more than A$500 for a birth. At that time the average fee for a home birth was A$1000. Tasmania was the only state to acquire ABS funding to set up a home birth service. This was made possible by the support (donations, cake-stalls, raffles etc.) of the Hobart Birth Support group. This project was only operative for 12 months and was not re-funded despite reported success on all levels.

South Australia has a project planned but, as with the midwives' teams, there is difficulty with the Nurses' Award system, which does not have contingency plans for midwives needing to work longer than 40 hours a week. Enterprise agreements are proving to be a quicker and more effective means of arriving at flexible time and work arrangements, than altering the industrial awards, much to the chagrin of some Unions.

A recent community trend to emerge is that more families are abandoning private health funds as the premiums continue to escalate for very small refunds. As more publicly (or Medicare) funded birth centres and midwives' clinics and teams open up, women are beginning to see that there is little benefit in having their own obstetrician, especially when only a small part of his fee will be reimbursed.

## NURSE PRACTITIONER PROVIDER NUMBERS

Since 1991 the NSW Department of Health has been wrestling with the problem of expanding nurses' roles without completely alienating medical practitioners. It is clear that nurses can give more accessible, more affordable and equally effective care to the public. Given the sums spent on educating nurses and the role they perform in situations where doctors are just not available, the state governments all recognise the need for change.

A first document *Nurse Practitioners in NSW, Stage 1* (New South Wales Department of Health 1991) set the scene for all nurses to gain accreditation through their appropriate speciality college or organisation, so that they may be awarded a 'provider number'. This provider number would allow nurses to order a range of pathology tests, and also to prescribe a range of drugs. These changes require alterations to the Health Act and the Nurses' Act.

Clearly this caused considerable consternation in the medical fraternity. The (then Deputy) Chairman of the Australian Medical Association (AMA) Brendan Nelson accused nurses of wanting to be doctors. Nurses and midwives were left with a vision of endless broken nights caused by the constant litigation which would follow the new powers. In NSW it was made clear that the industrial power and greater numbers of the NSW Nurses' Association would be required to accomplish this change for midwives.

Stage 2 (New South Wales Department of Health 1993) proposed four project models under the guidance of a corporate consultative company. The models call for nurses (my apologies to the reader, but midwives are *never* mentioned in this document) to be under the surveillance and supervision of doctors. With a large body of area health authorities to whom the nurses are accountable, a trial period of 1 year would test the efficacy of the plan. This is proposed despite the fact that nurses and midwives in remote and rural Australia, employed by the various state health departments, have been fulfilling the professional roles mentioned above for many years. Midwives regularly order vital tests for pregnant women and take responsibility for all the health care of their clients.

The only place deemed appropriate for midwives to take part in one of these trials must be within a hospital-based project. When the idea of provider numbers was first suggested there was only one example of the need, which also demonstrated the inequities of the current system: at home births and wherever independent midwives practise.

At a meeting to launch the Stage 2 document, a woman doctor representing the AMA, stated emphatically that even if all the models proved to be a resounding success, there was no guarantee that doctors would support the proposal for registered nurses to have provider numbers. Gruesome tales of the New Zealand economy, controlled as it is now by NZ midwives (*sic*) abound among Australian doctors, and they have managed to use these stories to terrorise the NSW Department of Health. The rest of the Australian states await NSW's results before they make a move in this direction.

## PROFESSIONAL INDEMNITY

For midwives to gain accreditation to both the ACMI and to individual hospitals, proof of professional indemnity must be shown. The independent midwives from NSW and Victoria were exceptionally proud of the indemnity policy drawn up with the assistance of an insurance broker through Lloyds of London. Initially it gave a cover of A$1 million charging premiums at a very reasonable level. This policy was available to all midwives in Australia and the clauses clearly define the role of the midwife as independent of doctors.

Despite this development, midwives felt considerable sadness and frustration that the Medical Defence Union of Australia recommended to its members that they should not support or give back-up services to independent midwives. Their information is that in litigation the doctor would be expected to take full responsibility for the actions of any individual midwife. Some hospital boards (for instance in NSW) insisted that the indemnity policy must be for at least A$5 million. The NSW Department of Health intervened and said that this was impossible and that the hospital boards must accept what the insurers had decreed.

Further negotiation with Lloyds of London resulted in a package whereby midwives may choose the level most appropriate to their needs, and Lloyds have agreed to an individual pay-out figure of A$5 million. Interestingly, since this flexible policy was introduced there has not been pressure on midwives to take the highest cover.

A landmark civil case was resolved out of court in 1993 in Sydney. A midwife, an obstetrician (who acted as back-up) and the hospital to which the woman was transferred in labour were sued. Though she was supported by the doctor in her actions, it was the insurance company of the midwife which was asked to pay out. This disproves the doctors' argument that a medical practitioner would always have to take responsibility in a court of law. Whilst the result was hard on the midwife, it verifies that the midwife may bear responsibility for being the primary care giver.

This case, as well as the fact that there has not been any pressure placed on midwives to take up the higher indemnity, demonstrated that it was not really a fear of litigation that caused doctors to erect barriers against midwives gaining visiting privileges, but the fear of a loss of clientele and a dislike of the appearance of midwives, within institutions, but obviously functioning as autonomous practitioners.

## EDUCATION: THE PRESENT AND THE FUTURE

Australia is at a point of great change in midwifery education. The system, which prevails in every state, insists that a midwife (according to the health departments and the ACMI definition) is a registered nurse with midwifery qualifications. Consequently many midwives who have trained in Europe and the Americas cannot register without first completing nurse training. Students applying for midwifery training must first be registered nurses. Until 1966 midwives could be trained by a direct entry course in Australia.

Nursing required a 4-year training until 1969 when it became a 3-year course. For many decades midwifery training was been a 1-year hospital certificate post-basic nursing course. By 1994 midwifery education was based in universities, with only one hospital in NSW still educating midwives through a hospital-based education system.

Attempts to introduce direct entry training at some universities have so far been unsuccessful. There appears to be a split among midwives about the appropriateness of direct entry training. Those who have achieved their status and recognition through the nursing path are reluctant to condemn the latter, or to see this route abandoned.

There are very few positions available for students to receive midwifery education. Similarly midwives who do not have a great deal of postgraduate experience are having difficulty in finding employment. This is most marked in NSW where the new legislation allows enrolled and registered nurses to act as midwives. The implications are clear: both midwifery and midwives have a very low priority.

In the State of Victoria, students undertaking their midwifery degrees are not required to find employment in a specified maternity unit. It is not clear how they will acquire clinical expertise. Under the former educational programmes, the hospital or area health service paid students for their hours of work within the hospital system. Now there is a range of options, from unpaid supernumerary positions to university schemes where the students begin to repay the cost once they are employed for a certain annual salary. The notion of owing allegiance to the person or body who pays the worker is a foreign one, as opposed to the clear situation in independent practice. The theoretical education of midwives is now most commonly conducted in universities, far removed from clinical surroundings. The very essence of midwifery, of a clinically oriented profession, 'with woman' first and foremost, appears to be obscured. During the clinical hours of a student's training, their experience is restricted by the medical model, despite the excellence and dedication of the midwifery tutors within the university campuses.

In response to this very fragmented educational system, the ASIM has presented a postgraduate course, in two consecutive years. Called the 'Midwives' Academy', independent midwives, childbirth educators and doctors offered to help midwives fulfil their role, so that they can function on their own responsibility and in any setting.

It is sad that many Australian midwives, training prior to the 1980s, did so in order that they could work in the bush, or on mission stations throughout the Third World, leaving their training institutions feeling confident that they were well prepared and well educated. In comparison with British- and European-trained midwives, Australian midwives have a strong ability to be innovative (caused by low budget hospital training), but they often demonstrate a lack of confidence in their own decision-making.

## THE CONSUMER VOICE

For a variety of reasons the power of the childbirth consumer appears to have disintegrated. Groups that were at their most vocal and active in the 1970s are now struggling for survival, as few people see the need for such lobbying mechanisms. The situation has not improved. The childbirth options open to women are not plentiful; the medical model has not changed. Lack of time, adherence to rosters and lack of respect for the childbirthing experience still rob most women of their most fulfilling moments in life.

One reason for the disintegration of the consumer voice, may be that: 'They have done their PR' as Beverley Beech of AIMS in the UK has put it. By giving women the option to have their baby at a birth centre, which their own Medicare dollar, amounting to 2% of wages, has paid for, women feel that they do have a choice. This choice, however, is made in the climate of few options rather than a wide and genuine range.

The realities of consumer choice are still very limited:

- Continuity of care is given only token consideration; women are still typically cared for by many different midwives and doctors during their pregnancy, labour and the birth.
- The definitions of a normal pregnancy and birth are so narrow that a small change in a woman's situation could deprive her of her ideal birth.
- Midwives providing care during labour may have to divide their time between two or more women, unable to give continuous care to any of them.
- Centres which have water baths do not allow birth in the bath as an option.
- Bedpans are still used, while en suite facilities remain unused.
- Labour is not allowed to extend longer than 12 hours.
- Women have limited choice of types of pain relief.
- Active management of the third stage is routine policy.
- Postnatal care is very limited, both in time (4–12 hours after a

normal birth, 36 hours after caesarean section) and available staff.

All these issues of hospital care demonstrate a lack of choice, and a failure to provide women with the care and nurturing they require during the events surrounding childbirth. It is observed that many doctors appear to find machinery more useful than holistic care, but this may be simply the result of not spending as much time as midwives allow for the one-to-one caring of women.

Other reasons why the consumer voice is heard less concern the financially insecurity and inequities in the health care system.

Another contributing factor is the increasing trend for women to return to work after childbirth. This is now occurring earlier than in previous decades, and as mothers leave their children in day care, so they lose the company and sense of purpose to be obtained from parenting groups.

Consumer groups feel, rightly, that they are helpless in the power struggles between the obstetricians and midwives. Midwives within institutions are restricted in their practice and do not develop confidence in making their own clinical judgements. Doctors state that they must make their own evaluations of the care needed. In emergency situations they frequently follow a course of action which is devoid of any personal knowledge of the woman's course of labour; this in turn can frustrate any planned midwifery care. It is my opinion that the fear of litigation, together with a type of 'jealousy' of the obvious bond that midwives develop from spending considerable periods of time with the women, inhibits trust and respect for the midwives, which results in the conflict and poor delivery of care. The woman is the one who suffers most in this environment, and those who wish to change the situation are rendered powerless.

There was a period between 1970 and 1985 when the Childbirth Education Association, Parent Centres Australia, and the Nursing Mothers' Association of Australia grew at an incredible pace. These organisations started with stencilled newsletters and kitchen table paste-ups and rapidly developed into producing more professional literature, with the advent of photocopiers, computers and laser printers. The need for the group effort of folding, sticking and pasting, to keep open the channels of communication, has gone and with it some of the recognition of communal activity. Couples attending such groups in the early 1970s could be counted on to give a few more years of service in appreciation of what they had gained. Now the sense of group identity is less and conflicting demands, such as work, brought about by the recession, mean that the strength and cohesiveness of the consumer groups has diminished.

There is much confusion and conflict about the Australian home birth outcome statistics of the early 1990s. Australian midwives have a sense of betrayal about the way the results of midwife-attended home births have been interpreted. This is one of the symptoms of the disease that has separated the midwives and the women they serve, preventing them from working together as they did in the past.

It is clear that some consumers have been swayed by the rhetoric of the medical profession, and though consumer involvement in committees such as the maternity services state reviews and organisations such as the ACMI, is token at best, they seem to be extremely grateful and not prepared to push for what the WHO (1985) sees as their rights:

... that people must be given the knowledge and influence to ensure that health developments are made not only for, but also with and by the people.

## CONCLUSION

Not the least of our difficulties has been the need for constant vigilance in challenging a series of 'regulations for midwives' which are designed to limit our practices. Birth centre protocols ensure that only women who fit into an ever narrowing range of 'normal' may use the facilities. These debatable and changeable lists of risks are seen as a means of harnessing midwives (in every setting) and carving out a clear 'doctor' only field which midwives must not overstep. The ACMI has fortunately, until now, rejected these moves. In addition the ACMI judged that restrictions placed on GPs by the Royal Australian College of Obstetricians and Gynaecologists (and at the time accepted by the Australian College of General Practitioners) would similarly not be in the best interest of their members.

Obstacles to the growth of the number of independent midwives concern issues of money and equitable care; the past role of midwives as handmaidens to doctors, and the fear of new challenges and responsibilities for all midwives that our very presence suggests. That the picture given here is one of struggle is perhaps not entirely fair to midwives who are just commencing their practice, and would see the job as one with more romance and satisfaction. Indeed this report fails to illuminate the absolute joy and rewards that working as an independent midwife can bestow. An independent midwife is constantly challenged to stretch her boundaries, and explore with women some of their most empowering and treasured moments in life.

This chapter has not shown the dedication of the Australian midwives travelling hundreds of miles into the bush, driving like madwomen lest the woman sorely needs a midwife's support, or the baby is born before arrival and there is a postpartum haemorrhage or a 'flat' babe; or the dedication of the midwives whose only access is over water, with the father coming to fetch the midwife and row her to the homestead before the valley is so flooded that access is impossible. These midwives have to face the worry of having to call in a helicopter if there is a need to transfer the woman in labour. They do this in the knowledge that they will 'get the flak' because they are prepared to give total allegiance to the women first, rather than to the system they would rather avoid.

Postnatal visits take a long time for these midwives, with a reluctance to leave as it is not possible to visit as often as is the custom in a city practice. They suffer the inhibition of trying to undertake telephone consultations that have to go through a main switchboard system or over the radio-operated phone. It is not easy to ask intimate questions about the woman's breasts or perineum, or even about the level of support when the whole district is listening in. Despite the difficulties, perhaps because of the challenges, the life of an independent midwife is one of great satisfaction.

This chapter has been written from the perspective of a NSW midwife. Although NSW has always had the largest number of home births and independent midwives, this does not mean that it always leads the other states in trends and developments. Australia is at present going through enormous change in its delivery of health care, not just maternity care. This chapter must be read with an awareness that the situation at the time of writing will alter over the next few months and years. The individuality of the states and their circumstances makes each state and area a unique entity, all of which add up to one very interesting conglomerate – Australia.

## ACKNOWLEDGEMENTS

I am indebted to the following women for their considerable knowledge of midwifery in their particular states, and their willingness to share it for the purposes of this chapter. Maria Nethecott of Victoria, Helen McDonald of Tasmania, Joy Argent of Northern Territory, Mary Murphy of Western Australia, Julie Pratt of South Australia, Denise Taynor of the Australian Capital Territory and Vicki Chan of Queensland. All are state representatives of the Australian Society of Independent Midwives.

REFERENCES

Flint C, Poulengeris P 1987 Know your midwife. Private publication
Medicare Benefits Review Committee 1986 The Layton Report. Australian Government Publishing Service, Canberra
Department of Health 1993 Changing childbirth Part 1. Report of the Expert Maternity Group (Chair J Cumberledge). HMSO, London
National Health and Medical Research Council 1994 Options for effective care in childbirth consultation document. Health Care Committee, NHMRC, January
New South Wales Department of Health 1991 Nurse practitioners in New South Wales: the role and function of nurse practitioners in New South Wales. Discussion paper prepared by The Task Force in Independent Nursing Practice in New South Wales in conjunction with the Nursing Branch, December
New South Wales Department of Health 1993 Nurse practitioners in New South Wales: the role and function of nurse practitioners in New South Wales. Discussion paper prepared by the Nursing Branch, June 1992
Rowley M 1994 Personal communication
Select Committee on Health 1992 Maternity services: second report of the House of Commons Health Committee (Chair N Winterton). HMSO, London
Willis E 1989 Medical dominance. Allen & Unwin, Melbourne
World Health Organization 1985 Targets for health for all. WHO, Geneva

# 4

# Independent midwifery in New Zealand

*Joan Donley*

## INTRODUCTION

October 1990 was a time of celebration for New Zealand midwives. After 20 years under direct medical supervision, they were given the opportunity to practise independently. This was the result of legislation initiated by the Labour Minister of Health, Helen Clark. The purpose of this legislation was to provide women with a wider choice of the underutilised options based on midwifery care, and to change women's perceptions of birth.

This effectively challenged the doctor's role as 'gatekeeper' and required the amendment of five Acts of Parliament and nine Regulations. These regulations in New Zealand are made by the Executive Council (i.e. the Governor-General and appointed ministers) and implement the purpose and policy of a statute, or law. As the regulations take effect by Orders-in-Council, they are outside the democratic process, and so are difficult to challenge in court. Consequently this change was particularly significant, and enabled midwives to prescribe medicines commonly used in pregnancy, order routine laboratory tests, make direct referrals to consultants and have access to public maternity hospital facilities on the same basis as general practitioners. It also established pay equity between doctors and midwives, as the latter could now claim on the doctors' more lucrative fee-for-service maternity benefit schedule.

Speaking to the Bill, Clark told MPs:

National home birth statistics in New Zealand reflect the benefits of commitment to natural childbirth and to continuity of care ... and the rejection of unnecessary interventions.

(Hansard 1990)

She went on to state that the challenge of the Bill was to ensure that the practices underlying the healthy statistics could be more broadly available to New Zealand women. Some of these statistics are shown in Table 4.1

## The move to independent practice

At first, only a few of the so-called 'relatively independent' domiciliary midwives (DMs) were prepared to make the quantum leap to independence. Two years later, approximately 50% of women opting for home birth chose midwifery-only care. However, out of 59 400 births in 1990, the 1037 home births amounted to only 2%.

**Table 4.1** The 1990 statistics of 1037 planned home births (source: New Zealand Homebirth Association)

| Outcomes | % |
| --- | --- |
| Transfer of mothers | 6.5 |
| Caesarean section | 1.8 |
| Forceps | 0.5 |
| Ventouse | 0.1 |
| Retained placenta | 1.0 |
| Transfer of babies | 1.2 |
| Postpartum haemorrhage | 3.4 |
| Mothers fully breast feeding | 98.2 |
| Perinatal mortality rate | 4.8/1000 |

## HISTORY OF MIDWIFERY CARE

The history of midwifery care in the previous 50 years had been one of the progressive medicalisation of childbirth. During this time women were conditioned to view pregnancy as an illness and birth as a medical crisis. The impact on midwives was that they were downgraded to acting as handmaidens of doctors. Despite the legality of midwifery, which had been recognised as part of the maternity system since 1904, the Nurses' Act of 1971 required every pregnant woman to be under medical supervision, and resulted in midwives becoming 'obstetric nurses' Specifically Section 52(a) made it an offence to practise 'obstetric nursing' unless a medical practitioner had undertaken responsibility for the care of the patient.

Midwives were so completely subsumed by nursing that there was not a murmur of protest at this legislation. A Midwives' Section (with about 200 members) was formed within the New Zealand Nurses' Association (NZNA) in 1972; this was, in fact, only used so that New Zealand could be a member of the International Confederation of Midwives.

### Medicalisation of birth

The 1970s in New Zealand, in common with a number of other countries, was a period in which the medicalisation of pregnancy was represented as progress. Much of this trend, in New Zealand, was based on the Postgraduate School of Obstetrics and Gynae-cology of the University of Auckland, and the associated clinical area of the National Women's Hospital (NWH). One of the most significant consequences of this approach was the regionalisation of services. This was in effect, a centralisation, which resulted in the closure of cottage hospitals in the rural and urban areas as well as of the private maternity hospitals.

### Home births

With the support of a strong feminist movement, many women rebelled against this increasing medicalisation and opted for home births, which were legal and were subsidised but at a low level. The fee-for-service of the domiciliary midwife was about 29% less than the salary paid to the government-funded hospital mid-wives. These home births were only legal if the women could find a GP courageous enough to 'undertake responsibility' for her care while the registered midwife carried out the 'obstetric nursing' allowed by the law (Nurses' Act 1971). For a brief period, one obstetrician undertook this responsibility – until he was threatened by his peers with the loss of his consultancy status. A similar situation which occurred in Australia is detailed in Chapter 3.

In spite of the unfavourable climate, in 1974, three domiciliary midwives set up in practice, two in Auckland on the North Island, and one 1500 miles away in Christchurch on the South Island. There were still a few GPs who would provide the necessary 'medical supervision' despite peer pressure. Even a few births outside hospital control, however, threatened the interests of both the medical and nursing professions. A Homebirth Support Group was set up in 1976, in Christchurch, to support their midwife working in isolation.

## New Zealand Homebirth Association

The formation of the Homebirth Association in Auckland in 1978, by a group of parents, was a political move to protect the home birth option. Starting with a membership of 150, it became a national organisation within 2 years, the NZHBA. Despite dependence on subscriptions, donations and voluntary labour, it was responsible for effecting many positive changes in the hospital system. By 1986 the ability of the homebirth movement as a 'pressure group . . . to make some headway against the medical establishment demonstrated their growing influence' (Minister of Health 1986), as was officially acknowledged.

The formation of the Homebirth Association prompted an immediate response from the Department of Health in which health professionals were advised to be more flexible in order: 'to counter this move away from our hospitals [to] protect the lives the IQs of our future citizens' (Maternity Services Committee 1979).

The Medical Council of the New Zealand Medical Association (NZMA), in conjunction with the Board of Health, established the Obstetrics Standards Review Committee to monitor standards, in particular those of GPs covering for home births.

## Maternity Services Committee

Practising outside the medical hierarchy, subject only to supervision of the Medical Officer of Health, domiciliary midwives were seen to be 'relatively independent'. The following year 1980, the NZNA drafted a policy statement on home confinement recommending standards. This was submitted to the Maternity Services Committee (MSC), adviser to the Board of Health on all matters regarding maternity care.

The MSC, a committee of 14, seven of whom were obstetricians, responded by setting up a survey of maternity care in the home. With a falling birth rate (from 62 050 live births in 1970 to 50 901 in 1980) the total of 1159 births between 1974 and 1980 (Cooper et al 1981) attended by fewer than 12 domiciliary midwives was seen as a dangerous midwifery precedent.

# MIDWIFERY TRAINING AND PROFESSIONAL STATUS

## Midwifery option of the Advanced Diploma of Nursing

By now the NZNA had made considerable progress in establishing the concept of the generalist 'family health' nurse who would provide continuity of care from birth to the menopause. The 6-month 'hands-on' midwifery training at the St Helens hospitals, established in the 1904 Midwives' Registration Act to train and register midwives to provide maternity care for the 'deserving poor', was terminated in 1979. The replacement was an 8–10 week 'midwifery option' within the Advanced Diploma of Nursing, which commenced in 1978 in several polytechnics.

New Zealand nurses responded to this change by going to Australia and the UK to gain a midwifery qualification. Consequently, of the 206 midwives registered by the Nursing Council in 1986, 177 (86%) had gained their qualification overseas and only 29 were graduates of the Advanced Diploma of Nursing. (Nursing Council of New Zealand 1987)

By 1981, the predominantly hospital-based midwife members of the Midwives' Section of the New Zealand Nursing Association were becoming critical of the nursing orientation of their nurse-midwife leaders. They came out in support of the domiciliary midwives who were challenging further NZNA recommendations to place them under obstetrician/hospital control (New Zealand Nursing Association 1981).

## Supervision by nurses

The next step was the Nurses' Amendment Act of 1983 which enabled any registered nurse to carry out or to supervise 'obstetric nursing'. By this time, 99% of births were in hospital under medical control, and obstetric nurses, the medical handmaidens, were the preferred health professionals.

The dismayed members of the NZNA National Midwives' Section prepared a submission for the Nurses' Amendment Bill 1983 Select Committee, but the NZNA National Executive would not permit it to be presented as it was based on the ICM definition of a midwife, which differed from the NZNA definition. The 12-member NZNA National Executive had three midwife members who represented midwifery as a specialised branch of nursing. Within the organisation as a whole, there were 20 000 nurses compared with 600 midwives.

Eventually, in 1985 the members of the Midwives' Section managed to have the ICM definition adopted at NZNA conference.

## Midwives united

The result of the Nurses' Amendment Bill 1983, was that hospital and domiciliary midwives united to save midwifery as a profession in its own right. They were supported by the home birth consumers. These efforts were also facilitated by the election of a Labour Government in 1984 which was supportive of both home births and midwifery.

In 1987 the Cartwright Inquiry into the treatment of cervical cancer at the National Women's Hospital raised the issues of patients' rights and informed consent at a national level. On the eve of the publication of the Cartwright Report, in August 1988, New Zealand midwives formed the New Zealand College of Midwives (NZCOM) to speak for midwives on all midwifery matters.

In accordance with the Cartwright recommendations and those of the World Health Organization (WHO 1985) the NZCOM included consumers as members and on its executive. This

**Table 4.2**   Midwives practising in New Zealand 1986

| Category | Age | | | | |
| --- | --- | --- | --- | --- | --- |
| | 19–29 | 30–49 | 50–59 | 60 + | Not recorded |
| Midwife | 2 | 107 | 55 | 11 | 1 |
| General/obstetric | 234 | 1709 | 672 | 126 | 98 |
| Comp/midwife* | 17 | 17 | — | — | 1 |
| Bridging** | 9 | 28 | 26 | 5 | 6 |
| Total | 262 | 1861 | 753 | 142 | 106 |
| % | 8.4 | 59.5 | 24.1 | 4.5 | 3.5 |

* When nursing training was transferred from hospitals to polytechs in 1984, the product was known as the 'comprehensive' nurse, who could function as a beginning practitioner in any health care system. Prior to this, the hospital graduate as a beginning practitioner could function only in the clinical area appropriate to her registration, e.g. psychiatric, psychopaedic, obstetric.
** The 'bridging' programmes were an interim measure to permit the hospital trained nurses to become registered comprehensive nurses.

eventually brought NZCOM into conflict with the ICM constitution, which specifies that member organisations must only consist of midwives.

With the formation of the NZCOM, the Midwives' Sections of the NZNA were dissolved. With the midwives now united in a single organisation, the struggle to upgrade midwifery education continued. Not only was there was a serious shortage of midwives (3124 registered practising midwives in 1986) but also 28.6% of them were over 50 years old (Table 4.2, Fig. 4.1).

An official evaluation of the 'midwifery option' of the Advanced Diploma in Nursing found that both the theoretical and clinical components were deficient. (Department of Education 1987). Together, consumer groups and midwives publicised the ICM recommendation of 35 midwives/1000 births and emphasised that New Zealand was 720 midwives short while Australia accused New Zealand of draining Australian health dollars to train midwives (Peters 1986).

## Separate midwifery education

The Departments of Education and Health established a working party of midwifery tutors and practising midwives to develop national guidelines for a 1-year separate midwifery education.

The NZCOM representatives ensured that the course was based

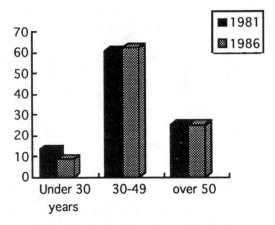

**Figure 4.1** Percentage of registered midwives in three age bands in 1981 and 1986 (Bazley 1986 and Department of Health 1986).

on the ICM definition of a midwife, to the alarm of the NZ Medical Association which realised the significance of training midwives to be independent practitioners. It commissioned a legal assessment of the course which confirmed it worst fears. For example:

> the structure . . . is clearly directed to a 'stand alone' responsibility for the patients, and there is no 'normal' doctor/nurse structure in existence.                    (Mazengarb 1989)

This was seen as 'exposing doctors' to an unacceptable professional position'.

Despite this opposition, courses commenced in February 1989 in different polytechnics which between them had approximately 100 registered nurses as students. The already established Government funding for 'bridging programmes' which was no longer required for the polytechnic training of the comprehensive nurses was transferred to provide capital equipment, infrastructure and tutors. Payment of student fees was often assisted by hospital boards which paid staff nurses partial or full pay in return for a guarantee to work for 2 years post graduation.

## PREGNANCY: A NORMAL PROCESS

Another important milestone in 1989 was the publication of a discussion document which was the result of 2 years of consultation with doctors, midwives and consumers. The document from the Department of Health (1989), *Care in Pregnancy and Childbirth*, was seen as a victory, as it acknowledged that pregnancy and childbirth are part of the normal life experience of women. The extent of this victory is only appreciated when it is realised that this was the first time since 1922 that the Department of Health officially agreed that these were normal processes.

This was also a first attempt at establishing national guidelines 'for the development of policy for safe options for low risk pregnancy' and at ensuring that women had choice and a voice in their care (Department of Health 1989).

## NURSES' AMENDMENT ACT

The next development in 1989 was the presentation of the Nurses' Amendment Bill to Parliament during November. This was the legislation which allowed midwives to practise independently.

Although the medical opposition to the Bill appeared to address the issue of safety, the real concerns were those of economics and territory. The New Zealand Medical Association, the College of General Practitioners, the Royal New Zealand College of Obstetrics and Gynaecology and the Medical Women's Association all voiced strong concerns about safety, the adequacy of midwifery training, and accountability in relation to independent midwifery. Submissions to the Select Committee suggested women should have access to compensation for midwifery misadventure. It was argued that the doctor was the obvious and necessary referral point, so all pregnant women should have a medical assessment with referral to a midwife as appropriate. Under the banner of competence, the midwives' right to prescribe such items as iron pills, antacids, laxatives and antifungal preparations was questioned, as this could extend to full prescribing rights.

## CONTROLS OVER MIDWIVES: NATIONAL PROTOCOLS

### Neonatal death at home

A few months after the passage of 1990 Act there was a neonatal death at home, several hours after an uneventful labour and normal birth attended by a midwife. Although New Zealand's foremost neonatal pathologist testified at the inquest that such unexplained deaths do regrettably occur even in hospitals, and in circumstances where the best technology is available, (Becroft 1991) the coroner concluded that: the greatest fault . . . is that the law permits home births to take place in the presence of a sole practitioner (Nelson Evening Mail 1991).

He called on the Minister of Health of the new national Government (elected October 1990) to review the law allowing midwives to deliver a baby without a doctor's supervision.

### Judicial review

The New Zealand College of Midwives felt the coroner's criticisms attacked the integrity of the profession. The College supported the midwife involved by applying for a judicial review in the High Court in order to provide a public forum in which to challenge the coroner's views free from the constraints of defamation laws.

This procedure was undertaken even though lawyers advised that a judicial review is concerned with the decision making process rather than the decision. This was reflected in a reserved judgement a year later in which the judge criticised the coroner but found in his favour.

## Arguments for control

The case mentioned above and a previous one were used to try to tighten controls over midwives, even though the conditions were different; one was a home birth and in the other the mother had been transferred and the birth occurred under medical supervision.

The earlier case involved a woman expecting her third child who was transferred from home with cervical dilatation of 6 cm, following the first sign of fetal heart rate irregularity. The hospital concerned had 8000 deliveries a year and at this time had a severe staff shortage (87 midwife vacancies), as well as problems of integrating two separate groups of staff with different attitudes. Following admission to hospital there was a 3-hour delay before the caesarean section was performed and subsequently the baby was diagnosed as having cerebral palsy. The health board acknowledged its responsibility for some of the delay.

These two cases were presented by the policy analysts in the Department of Health as 'potentially contributing to poor outcomes'. This argument was used to tighten up access agreements and justify recommendations for national protocols based on the task-oriented medical model (Project Report 1992).

## Opposition to protocols

The New Zealand College of Midwives (1992) in their submission to the Maternity Benefits Tribunal (see below) opposed:

protocols or proscriptive practice [as] not appropriate for practitioners required to exercise judgement . . . No woman, no labour and no baby are the same. It needs clinical judgement to ensure each mother and baby receive the best, the safest and most appropriate care.

## THE MATERNITY BENEFITS TRIBUNAL

This five-member tribunal was established by the Minister of Health in September 1992, at the insistence of the New Zealand Medical Association, as a result of the failure on the three parties (NZMA, NZCOM and Department of Health) to reach an agreement as to the scale of fees to be paid for midwifery and medical services.

Following the passage of the Nurses' Amendment Act 1990, the Government had been aware that there was a need for a more appropriate interpretation of the fee system, which had been' developed over the years through negotiation between the NZMA and the Department of Health, based on the medical model, and in the interests of the doctors. The 1990 Amendment made NZCOM a member of the negotiation committee.

A NZMA submission to the tribunal claimed it was not the role of a medical association to be negotiating benefits for independent midwives (Hill 1992). Although the Department of Health attempted to arrange meetings to examine the 'anomalies' which the Departmental advisers saw as beginning to affect the maternity services (Laracy 1992), no agreement could be reached as the NZMA boycotted these meetings.

## The 'schedule' (maternity benefit)

The real reason for the doctors' opposition was that pay equity struck at the very roots of the doctors' perceived and established status. Since the historic social legislation of 1939 which provided free, universal maternity and hospital care, New Zealand doctors collected the maternity benefit, based on a system known in New Zealand as 'the schedule'. In 1992 they demanded separate schedules, or scales of fees, for midwives, designed to put them back where they were seen to belong, i.e. as the doctors' handmaidens described by Rothman (1982) as 'physician extenders', as soyabeans are used to extend hamburger meat. A confidential report stated that 'separate schedules would send signals to consumers that one health professional was intrinsically more valued than the other'.

The NZMA claimed that their schedule was being used to 'piggy back' midwives (Laracy 1992) whom, they asserted 'merely sit with a woman'. They saw this as gross abuse of the system. Oddly, they did not consider that the generous benefit they collected for appearance at or after a birth, based on the unacknowledged work of the midwife, to be abuse of the system or that it was the midwives who were giving a 'piggy back' to the doctors.

## Payment of maternity benefit to doctors and domiciliary midwives

The 'schedule' or the fee-for-service maternity benefit, established in 1939, provides free maternity care for women, either in hospital under the care of a doctor of their choice, or at home under the care of a domiciliary midwife and/or doctor of their choice. While technically belonging to the woman, the fee is paid to the practitioners nominated by the woman. In the case of a home birth where both a midwife and a doctor attended, both were paid.

By 1989, through a process of regularly negotiated increments, this was set at $285 for the doctor for appearance at (or after) a birth, at home or in hospital. If the doctor was there for longer than one-and-a-half hours 'for medical reasons for special circumstances' a further $69.80 per half hour or part thereof thereafter was paid. This was known as 'prolonged attendance'.

In contrast the domiciliary midwives were paid on a fixed fee system decided by the Minister of Health for obstetric 'services rendered'. By 1989, however, through the perseverance of the New Zealand Homebirth Association, domiciliary midwives received $225 for care during labour and delivery up to 6 hours, plus $37.50 per hour thereafter.

## Abuses of the payment system

As mentioned above, after the passage of the 1990 Act 'anomalies' began to affect the maternity services, and failure to resolve these 'anomalies' resulted in abuses; for instance:

• Some obstetricians referred private patients to independent midwives so they could have one-to-one intrapartum care in hospital, subsidised by the schedule, at $69.80 per half hour after one-and-half hours. This not only duplicated costs and services, encouraged the obstetric model and fragmented care, it also maintained the doctor as gatekeeper and the midwife as handmaiden (Lovell & Virtue 1991).

• In the prevailing climate of 'market forces' area health boards also encouraged this practice. It relieved the salaried midwives in often understaffed delivery units, and shifted costs from the board's budget onto the schedule. This duplicated and increased costs (Department of Health 1992): for instance if the delivery unit was not busy it meant under-utilisation of salaried staff. Some obstetricians (Hutton 1992) claimed that midwives were allowed to hold onto relatively high risk women in open beds (those reserved for obstetricians' and GPs' private patients) threatening the viability of the obstetricians' closed units (i.e. clinic patients available for the training of medical students). GPs who did not do maternity care would prefer to refer a woman to the clinic rather than a rival doctor.

These anomalies also sowed discord among midwives on two levels:

• economic, because of the pay differential between independent and hospital (salaried) midwives;
• philosophical, as a number of midwives who felt safer with birth in hospital, under medical control, claimed to be 'independent'.

## The place of domiciliary midwives

Domiciliary midwives were aware that the only place a midwife is independent is in the community; outside both medical and hospital control. This, in turn, is dependent on a woman who wants to be in control of her own birthing process. This can only be achieved 'on her own turf' as the Kiwis say, be that her own home, Maori marae (community structure) or a free-standing community-controlled birth centre. Both doctors and midwives are entitled to the maternity benefit wherever the birth occurs. Women pay to have their babies in a private hospital/birth centre. The mothers also pay for the services of a private obstetrician although obstetricians also receive the maternity benefit.

## Increasing the maternity benefit

Despite calls for 'fiscal restraint' the doctors were lobbying for an increase in the maternity benefit (for doctors) which would cost the taxpayers $66m. Yet, they used the payment anomalies to try to cast doubt on the cost-effectiveness of midwives. A Wellington doctor is reported as saying:

At a time when the health service is so short of money and other services are being slashed, I think it is disgusting that so much money is being paid out to midwives.

(Thomas 1991)

Karen Guilliland, then NZCOM President countered that:

You cannot take seriously doctors who are going on about how 50 midwives are going to bankrupt the country while hundreds of doctors have been claiming from the Maternity Benefit, some for huge sums.

(Thomas 1991)

## Media coverage

In order to refocus attention onto safety issues, on the eve of the Tribunal, national TV launched a series of sensational programmes to show the dangers of the midwifery model. This was despite the Departmental confidential report (Department of Health 1992) which noted that the outcome of midwifery care for normal cases was of comparable quality to that provided by medical practitioners.

The report also noted that: Maternity services have a high public profile, especially when quality of care issues are involved, and went on to caution that there was a need for a 'careful public strategy to avoid misrepresentation of issues'.

## The tribunal proceedings

While the NZMA hired a Queen's Counsel as their legal representative at the Tribunal's preliminary public hearing (which lasted for 8 days) the NZCOM was brilliantly represented by Karen Guilliland, supported by a team of very articulate midwives who cross-examined the doctors and challenged both their evidence and their prejudices. Two previous Tribunals had been relatively cosy affairs between the NZMA and the Department of Health. This was the first time the doctors had been challenged by a third party and a female one at that.

The Tribunal completed its deliberations and recommendations in January 1993. The Minister of Health released the Department of Health final report in May 1993.

## The tribunal recommendations

### Payment issues

The principle of having one schedule was upheld. Under the outcomes-focused Public Finance Act (Department of Health 1993), outcomes of equal quality (Hyman 1993) must be paid for equally. The NZCOM expressed 'delight' that the principle of pay equity was upheld, but pointed out that the NZCOM supports a fee structure which encourages continuity of care, and the report neither challenged the status quo nor offered innovative solutions for an overall improvement to the maternity services funding arrangements (Department of Health 1993).

The prolonged attendance fee was to be replaced by a 'birth fee' of $313.60 payable for one-and-a-half hours before and during birth, plus a conduct of labour fee of $90.00 per hour after one-and-a-half hours. The birth fee could be claimed by two practitioners, but by only one practitioner if health board midwifery services were used. Most money is spent for normal birth in hospital. With 1653 registered midwives (out of a total of 3318) working in the obstetric/gynaecology field and 336 claiming the maternity benefit, it was expected that 11 000 of the estimated 53 500 births for 1992–1993 would involve either midwife 'shared care' or 'midwife only care'. The total cost on the current schedule was estimated to be nearly $82m (Department of Health 1993).

The Department granted a 10% increase in fees backdated 1 year (as opposed to the tribunal recommendation of a 26% increase backdated 2 years).

The NZMA felt this bore little resemblance to the tribunal recommendations.

Favouring a fee structure that encourages continuity of care, the

NZCOM felt that the relatively high fees for birth or caesarean section were inappropriate, placing too much value on techniques compared with the value placed on the skill and knowledge involved in the prevention of complications. The NZCOM favours an overall fee which recognises birth as a total event which each contact or service impacts on previous and future outcomes (Department of Health 1993).

### National protocols or guidelines

The issue of national guidelines was unresolved. The tribunal recommended that national guidelines be established for maternity care, although the NZMA had recommended national protocols. The NZCOM supported the concept of guidelines but not rigid protocols or standardised criteria.

The tribunal recommended that a body be established to set these guidelines. The Department of Health countered that a consensus conference would cost around $16 000 and suggested other existing bodies. This was 'totally unacceptable' to the NZMA which claimed that none of these 'bureaucratic bodies have the confidence of the profession'. (Department of Health 1993, Maternity Benefits Tribunal 1993).

## RESTRUCTURING OF THE HEALTH SERVICE

As the dust settles on the Maternity Benefits Tribunal–Department of Health recommendations, which became effective in August 1993, midwives and consumers are organising for the 'restructuring' of the entire health system. This restructuring which some midwives feel is, in fact, privatisation, came into force the month before the implementation of the maternity recommendations.

Four regional health authorities took over management of all health care in their own areas. They receive population-based funding and will contract services from providers. This, of course, has the potential to create divisions among various health professionals as they manoeuvre to cut costs to gain contracts.

## CONCLUSION

Not only must midwives stick together, they must also continually renew and reinforce their equal partnership with women. Now that health care is becoming a commodity and 'market forces' are added to modern obstetrics/medicalised childbirth, it is relevant to recall the claim of a New Zealand obstetrician that the three greatest threats to modern obstetrics are feminism, consumerism and midwives.

Midwives must assert their place in the care of childbearing women, with their slogan that had such an impact at the ICM 22nd Congress in Japan in 1990:

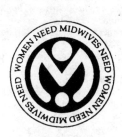

If we keep this as the central message, we will be able to meet these challenges and develop a maternity service which works primarily in the interest of mothers and their babies, supported by independent midwives.

REFERENCES

Bazley M 1986 Midwifery manpower in New Zealand in the 80s and 90s. Papers from Midwives Seminar, Auckland, 28 and 29 May 1982. Midwives Section, NZNA, Wellington, p 18–28

Becroft D 1991 Reported in the Nelson Evening Mail, 27 June 1991

Cooper D, Wittmer J, Pemberton J, Kennedy S, Taylor A 1981 Statistics for the Homebirth Association. Auckland Homebirth Association, Wellington, New Zealand

Department of Education 1987 An evaluation of the Advanced Diploma in Nursing courses. Research and Statistics Division, Department of Education, Wellington, New Zealand

Department of Health 1986 The Nursing workforce in New Zealand. Department of Health, Wellington, New Zealand, p 71

Department of Health 1989 Care in pregnancy and childbirth. Safe options for low risk pregnancy. Department of Health, Wellington, New Zealand

Department of Health 1992 Report on the review of the Maternity Benefit Schedule. Department of Health, Wellington, New Zealand

Department of Health 1993 Final report on the report and recommendations of the Maternity Benefits Tribunal. Department of Health, Wellington, New Zealand

Hansard 1990 Proceedings of 21 August 1990. Government Publication, Wellington, p 3677

Hill K 1992 Submission to Maternity Benefits Tribunal
Hutton J 1992 Submission to Maternity Benefits Tribunal
Hyman P 1993 Evidence in the report and recommendations of the Maternity Benefits Tribunal 1993
Laracy L 1992 Maternity fees dispute heads towards Tribunal. NZ Doctor 7 February, 1992
Lovell M, Virtue C 1991 Internal NZCOM document presented at Board of Management meeting. New Zealand College of Midwives, Wellington
Maternity Benefits Tribunal 1993 Report and recommendations 13 January 1993. Government publication, Wellington, New Zealand
Maternity Services Committee of the Board of Health 1979 Obstetrics and the winds of change. Government publication, Wellington, New Zealand
Mazengarb M 1989 Assessment of national guidelines for the training of midwives. Letter to the NZMA
Minister of Health 1986 Choices for health care: report of the health benefits review. Government publication, Wellington, New Zealand, p 56
Nelson Evening Mail 1991 Report 27 June 1991, p 1
New Zealand College of Midwives 1992 Submission to Maternity Benefits Tribunal, Government publication, Wellington, New Zealand
New Zealand Department of Statistics 1974–80. Annual reports. Government publication, Wellington, New Zealand
New Zealand Nurses' Association 1981 Policy statement on maternal and infant nursing. NZNA, Wellington
Nurses' Act 1971 Section 52(b) Government publication, Wellington, New Zealand
Nursing Council of New Zealand 1987 Annual Report. Government publication, Wellington, New Zealand
Peters M 1986 Unpublished paper presented to the NZ Midwives' Conference, Christchurch, September
Project Report 1992 Pregnancy and childbirth standards: protocols and access agreements. Department of Health, Wellington
Rothman B K 1982 In labour: women and power in the birthplace. Junction Books, London
Thomas M 1991 Midwives earn huge amount say doctors.
The Dominion (Wellington) 13 December
World Health Organization 1985 Appropriate technology for birth, Lancet 2 (8452): 436–437

# Midwifery education

## SECTION CONTENTS

# 5

# Midwifery graduates in the United Kingdom

*Jo Alexander*

## INTRODUCTION

I have been sporadically involved with moves to increase the availability of both graduate education in midwifery and graduate education for midwives since the early 1980s and I welcome this opportunity for reflection.

Presumably, as with nursing (MacGuire 1991), there are at least four pathways which could result in midwives holding both a degree and their professional qualification. There are:

- those who hold a degree before undertaking midwifery education
- midwives who subsequently undertake degrees
- those who gain their midwifery registration simultaneously with a degree in midwifery (whether through a preregistration or postregistration course), and potentially
- those who might gain midwifery registration simultaneously with a degree in an informing discipline such as psychology or sociology, but I am not aware there are currently even plans for such a course.

I have chosen to limit my discussion almost exclusively to the third pathway, as it seems likely that this will be the most important in terms of numbers. I have tried to investigate the probable validity of some of my beliefs concerning the benefits which could result from graduates in midwifery influencing the profession. Whilst I do not believe midwifery to be a branch of nursing, there are certainly areas of similarity between the two professions and so it seems suitable to examine the literature on nursing courses which lead to first registration at the same time as gaining a nursing degree, in order to try to identify some themes which may prove relevant to midwifery.

## THE IMPROVEMENT OF CLINICAL PRACTICE

The cornerstone of my belief in the desirability of graduate studies in midwifery is that they must surely improve the standard of clinical practice; if they do not benefit the clients, I can see little point in them.

One way in which one might expect the standard of clinical practice to be improved would be through the application of research findings, and the importance of this appears to be stressed more in undergraduate than in diploma level courses (Winson 1993). There has been a considerable increase in the volume of research relevant to midwifery practice published over recent years (Midwifery Research Initiative 1991), and one might assume that graduates, having been taught to read research critically, would be in a good position to promote any necessary changes in practice. One wonders if this has been the pattern following the introduction of nursing degrees and, more generally, what effect graduate education has on clinical practice.

### Comparisons of clinical abilities

Assessing the standard of an individual's clinical practice is always a difficult nettle to grasp and it seems (Bircumshaw 1989a) that there have been few British or American studies of undergraduate students which have tried to consider their clinical abilities. O'Brien (1984) describes a questionnaire survey of ward sisters who had had undergraduates allocated to their wards and they generally had a very high opinion of the students' abilities. There is also evidence (Waters et al 1972), based on short-term observation of staff nurses in the clinical setting and subsequent discussion with them, that baccalaureate nurses are more likely to consider the patient's psychological and social needs, and not to plan their nursing actions on physiological and physical considerations alone.

There appear to have been only two British studies which have tried to compare those undertaking (or who have undertaken) a Bachelor of Nursing (BN) course with those from a traditional course. Crow (1980) investigated whether 22 BN students, from two different universities, and 18 state registered nursing ('traditional') students, from two different teaching hospitals, differed in their ability to identify nursing problems from a nursing history and suggest nursing interventions. The students were tested (once only) after they had been on their course for 9 months, and their answers were compared with those produced by a panel of nurses. The relationship between thinking style and performance was also investigated. In addition, a group of educationalists involved with the undergraduate courses was compared with a group involved with the 'traditional' courses; the characteristics which they would encourage in their students were compared.

The BN students were significantly more likely ($p = 0.05$) to identify problems of a social nature than the 'traditional' students, and it was suggested that this might have been due to the greater tendency of their lecturers to encourage creative personality traits than that demonstrated by those who taught the 'traditional' students. A significant positive relationship existed between the respondents' ability to use divergent (as opposed to convergent) thinking and their ability to identify actual problems. There was a strong association ($p = 0.001$) between divergent thinking and an ability to suggest nursing interventions, and between divergent thinking and an ability to identify biological problems. Crow (1980) defines creative (divergent) thought as 'innovative, exploratory, venturesome . . . impatient of convention . . . attracted by the unknown and undetermined', and non-creative (convergent) thought as 'cautious, methodical, conservative . . . absorbs the new into the already known and expands existing categories in preference to devising new ones'. There was however no clear distinction between the thinking style of the BN and 'traditional' students! It would appear to be desirable to encourage divergent thinking.

The other British study (Bircumshaw 1988) is described later with some detail given of the midwifery results. She found few startling differences between the 19 BN graduates and the matched traditionally trained nurses whom she studied. It is perhaps a relief that she did find that the graduates considered themselves to be more competent at applying knowledge in the clinical situation than the non-graduates considered themselves to be. She came to the conclusion that more might be achieved if groups of graduates worked in association rather than in isolation and that such situations should be researched.

It is worth noting that neither of these studies involved observation of the subjects in the clinical situation. Bircumshaw's pilot study (Bircumshaw & Chapman 1988) included small scale non-participant observation, using activity analysis, but it gave little information about the way in which the subjects practised. She makes the point (Bircumshaw 1989a) that an appropriate and realistic assessment of clinical practice would probably require a more qualitative approach.

In 1982, Hayward argued that there should be differences between a nurse who entered the profession via a university and one trained traditionally; that the profession should be clear what differences it was aiming at, and that the differences should be clearly identifiable. He suggested that these differences should go far beyond those of knowledge levels. Unfortunately we still seem to have a long way to go, not least as regards investigating the differences.

It will therefore be important for research to be conducted to compare the clinical skills of graduate midwives with those of midwives educated through non-graduate courses (possibly both diplomate and non-diplomate). This research is needed not least to answer the questions of those who are sceptical (Jackson 1993) about the value of graduate preparation for midwives. Bircumshaw's survey (1989b), which explored the attitudes of senior nurses to the graduate nurses working within their localities, indicated that graduates may lack confidence, at least initially, and take longer to settle into their first staff nurse post than traditionally trained nurses. It would therefore seem desirable for such a comparison of clinical skills to be delayed until both groups of 'students' have been in post for at least 6 months.

## Using skills to their full potential

Graduate nurses (Bircumshaw 1989b) have commented that the

extent to which they can use their skills to 'practise differently' depends on the degree to which they are allowed and indeed expected to do so. It therefore follows that, for such a comparison to give an indication of the relative clinical value of the courses, the midwives must be practising in an area where each individual is encouraged to use their skills to their full potential. There seems never to have been any consensus about the role of the graduate in the nursing profession (Bircumshaw 1988, Morle 1988) and one can only presume that, in many circumstances, their skills must be underused as a result.

## Attitudes of colleagues

One factor that influences the extent to which individuals feel able to use their skills must surely be the attitudes of colleagues. It is well documented that undergraduate student nurses feel that they suffer resentment, suspicion, hostility and prejudice and are perceived as being different from 'traditional' student nurses (O'Brien 1984). Luker (1984) found that students reported that the experience was tantamount to being stigmatised. This was probably due (at least in part) to the trained staff feeling threatened by them, because they perceived the students as challenging the established 'moral order' that what counts is years of experience. Smithers & Bircumshaw (1988) considered that the passage of time had reduced this problem but Laurent (1991) indicates that undergraduate nurses are still having to cope with resentment from ward staff.

The stress caused to students by trying to be 'the same but different' (Bircumshaw 1988) appears to be very great. In addition, the processes to which they resort in order to gain acceptance, such as self-denigration and controlling the disclosure both of their undergraduate/graduate status and of their knowledge of the theoretical underpinnings of nursing practice (Luker 1984, Bircumshaw 1988), hardly sound conducive to producing an environment in which to advocate clinical change successfully. Indeed House (1975) indicates that undergraduates she interviewed considered that they would not be able to effect change until they had proved themselves to be 'good practitioners', and Smithers & Bircumshaw (1988) add that students must also be accepted as people before they can attempt even minor changes needed to implement what they have been taught.

This problem may not however be limited to graduates, for in her questionnaire study of both graduates and non-graduates Bircumshaw (1988) found that the latter also said that they had tried unsuccessfully to promote change! Unfortunately, in the past midwives have not been renowned for valuing the skills that postregistration students bring with them; rather, the 'can you take a blood pressure?' syndrome has been evident (Cowan 1986).

In the future therefore it is vital that we, as midwives, have enough genuine interest in the welfare of our clients, enough confidence in the overall quality of our practice and in the value of what we teach our students, and enough generosity of spirit to get our professional subculture right.

## The theory–practice divide

Smithers & Bircumshaw (1988) argue that undergraduate courses provide the potential for an even greater gulf between theory and practice than do 'traditional' courses.

Turton (1985) suggests there is:

a fundamental difference in the university and nursing approach to criticism, questioning and controversial argument. In a university student these are seen as positive. In nursing they are still widely regarded as negative.

The resulting conflict has been documented by many authors (House 1975, O'Brien 1984, Smithers & Bircumshaw 1988). When the midwifery undergraduate course in Oxford was designed, a deliberate effort was made to minimise this conflict by trying to ensure that the organisation of the clinical environment allowed both discussion and challenge, and the role of lecturer-practitioner was developed (Page & Healey 1990). Certainly one would wish university lecturers to be 'visionary' and yet to have at least one foot firmly planted in clinical reality, so that graduates may avoid the 'reality shock' on qualification which has been so clearly described (Kramer 1974, Simpson 1979).

## Quality assurance

The principles of quality assurance should surely be included in an undergraduate programme, and therefore one would expect graduates to influence the standard of midwifery practice through this medium. Recent research has indicated that, unfortunately, in midwifery there is relatively little activity related to quality assurance when compared to nursing, and what there is was considered to be half-hearted (Dawson 1992). This is especially topical as the second report of the Health Committee (Select Committee on Health 1992) has stressed that midwives 'have a right to develop and audit their own professional standards'.

## RESEARCH BY MIDWIVES

It seems to me that an increase in undergraduate midwifery courses should ultimately lead to an increase in the amount of research being conducted by midwives and that this should lead to improved clinical practice.

There is certainly scope for more midwives to become involved in research. Hicks (1991), in a national survey of 250 randomly selected nurses and midwives, found that only 8% of midwives had carried out independent research which was not part of course requirements. It is encouraging that Akinsanya (1994) thinks that one of most important results of the setting up of undergraduate nursing courses in the UK has been a rapid growth in the development of nursing research.

However I am not alone (Renfrew & Sleep 1992, personal communication) in having grave doubts about undergraduate students undertaking research involving clients. The students' limited understanding of research methods and their range; the very restricted time available to prepare a proposal, negotiate access, gain ethical approval, carry out data collection with an adequate sample size and complete the research process; the difficulties of providing adequate and appropriate supervision, and the sheer weight of student numbers, all militate against the conduct of client–based research at this level. Added to this, the Royal College of Physicians (1990) considers that 'research that causes inconvenience to subjects . . . without producing useful or valid results, is unethical' and most undergraduate research is likely to fall into this category. Research can be taught in a variety of lively and interactive ways without requiring access to clients (Clark & Sleep 1991).

In her survey of nurses who had graduated from Hull at least 5 years earlier, Kemp (1990) found that eight students (12.5% of respondents) gave research as their principal occupation and that many others identified a smaller research commitment within their main role. Like Morle (1989), she also found that graduates tend to embark on a further 'course' within 2 years of graduation, some of these being at higher degree level. It would seem likely therefore that, in the fullness of time, midwifery graduates will add to the body of knowledge on which we base the advice we give to clients.

It appears, unfortunately, that many midwives feel that they are being urged to carry out research without first gaining a firm grasp of research principles and the methodologies they wish to use. If this is the case, it must surely be a grave mistake, and may in part explain Hicks' finding (1992) that midwives were significantly more likely to rate as inferior a paper that they believed was written by a midwife than a paper that they believed was written by an obstetrician, even when the attribution was reversed for half the sample!

There is certainly a need for midwives to carry out research as they 'ask different questions' (Chalmers 1992). However, it is essential that they are properly trained and supervised, so that they produce good quality research which, hopefully, will be valued by the profession.

## CAREER PATHS OF GRADUATES

In her review of the literature about the career patterns of British nursing graduates, MacGuire (1991) calls for a meta-analysis of the various studies that have been conducted, and indeed this seems long overdue. However, even without this analysis some trends can be identified, and she states that most students seem to move into clinical posts on graduation and that they do not seem to have an 'accelerated career path' or to move away from nursing. These findings from earlier surveys received further support from a follow-up study of 214 nurses who graduated from the University of Glasgow during the years 1982–1990 (Smith 1993). Howard & Brooking (1987) and Kemp (1990) found that those who had graduated a few years previously tended to have an increasing orientation towards community care.

### Professional autonomy

In addition to the tendency towards community care Kemp (1990) identified a trend towards posts 'perceived to have more autonomy, social hours of work and opportunities for self-development'. This characteristic of an orientation towards professional autonomy was demonstrated by Murray & Morris (1982) to be considerably more prevalent among senior baccalaureate students than among those undertaking other kinds of nursing programme. Bircumshaw (1988) also found from her questionnaire completed by graduate and non-graduate nurses, that the graduates tended to score more highly for their interest in nursing autonomy and advocacy, patients' rights and rejection of traditional role limitations. The difference however was not significant.

In a questionnaire survey of 1000 randomly selected members of the Royal College of Midwives, Buchan & Stock (1990) found that 55% of respondents considered community midwifery to be more likely to enable practitioners to use their initiative than hospital-based midwifery, nursing or health visiting. Considerably more of the community midwives questioned considered the ability to use their initiative as an important factor when choosing a career than did the hospital-based midwives. Thus it seems likely that a large proportion of midwifery graduates will ultimately work as community midwives or as independent practitioners and, despite the fact that the first cohort graduated in 1994, there is already evidence of such career plans (Cardale 1992).

However, given the Health Committee recommendations (Select Committee on Health 1992) that most midwives should have their own caseload and that there should be 'midwife-managed maternity units', and the subsequent recommendations of the Expert Maternity Group of the Department of Health (1993), this trend may prove to be less marked than it might otherwise have been.

In theory one might expect that graduates would tend to find their strong desire for professional autonomy frustrated in many traditional nursing jobs and therefore be likely to leave the profession. However (as discussed above) this does not appear to happen.

## Recognition of the skills of graduates

Unlike the Civil Service, nursing has no separate career path for graduates and it must surely be significant, as MacGuire (1991) has pointed out, that even a degree in nursing itself is not a registrable qualification in the United Kingdom. The current grading definitions (Review Body for Nursing Staff, Midwives, Health Visitors and Professions Allied to Medicine 1988) do not provide grounds for accelerated progress simply on the basis of having a degree; higher grading is dependent upon increasing responsibility for clinical work or its management, and the education and supervision of others. Morle (1989) suggests that clinical regrading has missed an important opportunity to give special recognition to graduates and there is some feeling among senior nurses that graduates should have higher salaries (Bircumshaw 1989b).

Bircumshaw herself, however, raises the question of whether it should be 'merit' that attracts financial reward, rather than just academic status, and once again the issue of defining and determining merit presents itself. One is brought back to her point that if graduates are to exercise their analytical skills these must be recognised, valued and their use encouraged.

The key to this lies in the support of those in senior positions, some of whom, on the basis of evidence collected by Bircumshaw (1989b), appear in the past to have been unimaginative and ill-informed. It seems very sad that nursing graduates do not rise to senior positions more quickly and in fact seem slow to seek promotion (Altschul 1983, Howard & Brooking 1987). Reid et al (1987) even reported that 42% (21/50) of respondents had experienced some negative reaction to their graduate status since finishing the course, some of this being from those in positions of professional authority.

Valerie Tickner (1992) feels that midwifery graduates should be valued for the different perspective and additional useful skills that they will bring to the profession but that it is important that this valuing does not become obsequious in nature.

## PERCEPTIONS OF 'PRACTICE STYLE' OF GRADUATES AND NON-GRADUATES

One study of particular interest to midwives is that conducted by Bircumshaw (1988) in which she compared the 'practice style' of 19 BN graduates from the University of Wales with that of non-graduates. Five of the graduates were practising as midwives.

Each graduate was matched with a non-graduate on the basis of age, sex, level of education before entering nurse education, experience since qualifying as a nurse, postregistration qualifications and present work environment. Their images of nursing, midwifery or health visiting, the personal importance which they attached to aspects of these images and their attitudes towards various aspects of their role were investigated by way of questionnaires. Using a card sort, they described the elements which they incorporated into their practice and rated their levels of competence and knowledge. (Further details of the instruments are given in Bircumshaw & Chapman 1988.)

While it must be remembered that the graduates had a degree in nursing and not midwifery, and that the sample size was very small, five graduate midwives being compared with four non-graduate midwives with one of the non-graduates being matched with two graduates, this study provides a unique opportunity to gain some idea of how graduate education may affect a midwife's perceptions and possibly practice.

## Characteristics of midwifery

When asked to indicate from a list which characteristics (not necessarily having their approval) corresponded to their 'picture' of midwifery, there were some noticeable differences between the graduate and the non-graduate midwives. More graduates ($n = 5$) attributed the following characteristics to midwifery than non-graduates ($n = 4$):

- solid intellectual content (4 vs 0)
- clear-cut lines of authority (4 vs 0)
- human drama and excitement (3 vs 1)
- high technical skill (4 vs 2).

Conversely, more non-graduates thought that emotional control and restraint characterised midwifery than did graduates (3 vs 0). There were also differences when the subjects were asked to indicate which characteristics, from the same list, were important to them personally, whether or not the characteristic was thought to be connected with midwifery. More of the graduates considered the following to be important than the non-graduates:

- human drama and excitement (3 vs 0)
- high technical skill (2 vs 0)
- ability to innovate in the solution of problems (5 vs 2)
- exercise of imagination and insight (4 vs 2).

## Application of knowledge, research and interpersonal skills

Graduate midwives considered themselves less likely to base practice on a medical model than non-graduates and less likely to adopt a task-orientated approach.

There were also some noticeable differences in the frequency with which the groups considered themselves likely to apply certain 'types' of knowledge to the practice situation. Three of the graduates ($n = 5$) considered they applied knowledge of behavioural sciences 'most of the time' as opposed to one non-graduate ($n = 4$); this may be at least partly explained by the fact that non-graduates had a poorer perception of their level of knowledge in this area. Interestingly all four of the non-graduates reported applying knowledge of nursing/midwifery/health visiting theories 'most of the time' as opposed to one of the graduates.

Two of the non-graduates reported applying research findings to practice 'most of the time' whereas no graduate felt that they did this, two feeling that they did so 'sometimes' and three 'never'! The reasons given, in general, by the graduates for not implementing research were lack of time, incentive and encouragement, whereas those given by non-graduates were lack of knowledge and awareness. It is perhaps some small comfort that all of the graduates felt their competence to apply research findings to practice settings to be above average. (Three of the non-graduates felt their competence in this area to be 'average' and one 'below average'.)

In addition to this, Bircumshaw has subsequently commented (1992) that a possible explanation for her finding is that the graduates were aware of much more research relevant to their clinical practice than the non-graduates were, and thus more aware of how much of it they failed to implement.

Finally, all of the graduates felt that they used interpersonal skills 'most of the time' when practising, as opposed to only two of the non-graduates.

## CONCLUSION

Obviously, for the reasons discussed, the above findings can be considered no more than interesting. For myself, however, the merest suggestion of the following is enough to make me feel that we should go forward with courage and determination.

An increase in the number of graduate practitioners could result in greater

- recognition of the intellectual content of midwifery
- application of knowledge from the behavioural sciences
- interest in innovative and imaginative problem-solving
- valuing of interpersonal skills,

and it could result in reduced

- feelings that midwifery is characterised by emotional control and restraint
- use of a medical model of practice
- use of task-orientated approach.

There are many other issues to be considered:

- Given the great emphasis being placed on the assessment of academic attainment, what criteria are being developed for assessing clinical skills?
- Do we know what constitutes 'a good practitioner' anyway; surely there is a need for a qualitative study?
- How can we most effectively bridge the theory–practice divide?
- Will graduate status alter the midwife–doctor relationship?
- Will graduate status help midwives to empower their clients to obtain the type of care they want and, when necessary, to act as their clients' advocates?
- Will women have more confidence in the skills of midwives who are graduates and be less convinced of the need to see a doctor?
- Will graduate status encourage women to view midwives as being elitist and therefore as less approachable authority figures?
- Should we aim for an all-graduate profession, and would the price of this be a reduction in the number of midwives employed and an increase in the number of health care assistants?

I suggest that the fundamental issue is this: the nursing profession has never been clear about the 'special skills' that it expects its graduates to have; it has often hampered its graduates as they try to apply research findings in the clinical setting and generally try to use their 'special skills', and it has not adequately investigated the clinical outcomes of graduate education. As the midwifery profession starts along this road, we have the advantage of seeing where nursing has stumbled; it will be even more reprehensible if we slip into the same pitfalls.

## ACKNOWLEDGEMENTS

This chapter has been developed, with kind permission, from a guest editorial in the Journal of Advanced Nursing (Alexander 1993). The comments of the following are also gratefully acknowledged: Denise Bircumshaw, Elaine Healey, Mary Renfrew, Sarah Roch, Jennifer Sleep and Valerie Tickner.

REFERENCES

Akinsanya J A 1994 Making research useful to the practising nurse. Journal of Advanced Nursing 19: 174–179
Alexander J 1993 Degrees in midwifery: aspirations and realities. Journal of Advanced Nursing 18: 339–342
Altschul A T 1983 Nursing and higher education. International Journal of Nursing Studies 20(2): 123–130
Bircumshaw D 1988 A study of the practice style of graduate and non-graduate nurses/midwives/health visitors. Unpublished Master of Nursing thesis, University of Wales (College of Medicine), Cardiff, p. 2, 103, 106, 119, 120, 170, 174, 210, 212
Bircumshaw D 1989a How can we compare graduate and non-graduate nurses? A review of the literature. Journal of Advanced Nursing 14: 438–443
Bircumshaw D 1989b A survey of the attitudes of senior nurses towards graduate nurses. Journal of Advanced Nursing 14: 68–72
Bircumshaw D 1992 Personal communication
Bircumshaw D, Chapman C M 1988 A study to compare the practice style of graduate and non-graduate nurses and midwives: the pilot study. Journal of Advanced Nursing 13: 605–614
Buchan J, Stock J 1990 Midwives' careers and grading. Institute of Manpower Studies report no 201. University of Sussex, Brighton, p 65, 68
Cardale P 1992 Midwifery – the direct route. Nursing Times 88 (13): 58–60
Chalmers I 1992 Evidence cited in Select Committee on Health 1992, para 427
Clark E H, Sleep J 1991 The what and how of teaching research. Nurse Education Today 11: 172–178
Cowan L 1986 Training for midwifery in the 1980s. Midwife, Health Visitor and Community Nurse 22(11): 384–385
Crow J 1980 Effects of preparation on problem solving: an investigation into student nurses' ability to identify problems and to suggest nursing interventions. Royal College of Nursing, London, p 16, 84, 85, 86
Dawson J 1992 Quality assurance in health care – the perception of nurses, midwives and managers. Unpublished PhD thesis, University of Southampton, Southampton
Expert Maternity Group of the Department of Health 1993 Changing childbirth. HMSO, London
Hayward J 1982 Universities and nursing education. Journal of Advanced Nursing 7: 371 – 377

Hicks C M 1991 Midwives' and nurses' attitudes to research. Unpublished report, School of Continuing Studies, University of Birmingham, Birmingham

Hicks C 1992 Research in midwifery: are midwives their own worst enemies? Midwifery 8: 12–18

House V G 1975 Paradoxes and the undergraduate student nurse. International Journal of Nursing Studies 12: 81–86

Howard J M, Brooking J I 1987 The career paths of nursing graduates from Chelsea College, University of London. International Journal of Nursing Studies 24(3): 181–189

Jackson K 1993 Midwifery degree programmes: who benefits? British Journal of Midwifery 1(6): 274–275

Kemp J 1990 Career patterns of graduates in nursing. Nursing Standard 5(4): 36–39

Kramer M 1974 Reality shock – why nurses leave nursing. C V Mosby, St Louis

Laurent C 1991 A matter of degree. Nursing Times 87(39): 34–35

Luker K A 1984 Reading nursing: the burden of being different. International Journal of Nursing Studies 21(1): 1–7

MacGuire J M 1991 Nurses with degrees in the United Kingdom: careers and contributions and challenges. Journal of Advanced Nursing 16: 625–627

Midwifery Research Initiative 1991 MIRIAD – Midwifery research database. National Perinatal Epidemiology Unit, Oxford, p 12

Morle K 1988 Recruitment . . . the graduate nurse. Nursing Education Today 8: 39–42

Morle K 1989 Where nursing education should be based. Nursing Standard 3(25): 25–28

Murray L M, Morris D R 1982 Professional autonomy among senior nursing students in diploma, associate degree, and baccalaureate nursing programs. Nursing Research 31(5): 311–313

O'Brien D 1984 Evaluation of an undergraduate nursing course. Journal of Advanced Nursing 9: 401–406

Page L, Healey E 1990 Midwifery by degree: changes in education and service in Oxford. Midwife, Health Visitor and Community Nurse 26(10): 364–365, 370

Reid N G, Nellis P, Boore J 1987 Graduate nurses in Northern Ireland: their career paths, aspirations and problems. International Journal of Nursing Studies 24(3): 215–225

Renfrew M J, Sleep J 1992 Personal communication

Review Body for Nursing Staff, Midwives, Health Visitors and Professions Allied to Medicine 1988 The fifth report on nursing staff, midwives and health visitors, CM360. HMSO, London, p 44–48

Royal College of Physicians 1990 Guidelines on the practice of ethics committees in medical research involving human subjects, 2nd edn. Royal College of Physicians, London, p 3

Select Committee on Health 1992 Maternity services: second report of the House of Commons Health Committee (Chair Winterton N) HMSO, London

Simpson I H 1979 From student to nurse – a longitudinal study of socialization. Cambridge University Press, Cambridge p 105

Smith L 1993 A follow-up study of the Bachelor of Nursing graduates 1982–90, University of Glasgow, Scotland. Journal of Advanced Nursing 18: 1840–1848

Smithers K, Bircumshaw D 1988 The student experience of undergraduate education: the relationship between academic and clinical learning environments. Nurse Education Today 8: 347–353

Tickner V 1992 Personal communication

Turton P 1985 Some awkward questions. Nursing Times 81(23): 22

Waters V H, Chater S S, Vivier M L, Urrea J H, Wilson H S 1972 Technical and professional nursing: an exploratory study. Nursing Research 21(2): 124–131

Winson G 1993 Comparing degree and diploma courses. Senior Nurse 13(5): 37–41, 44

# 6

# The education of midwives in Australia: current trends and future directions

*Lesley Barclay*

## INTRODUCTION

It is pertinent to review the issue of the educational preparation of midwives in Australia because this is a time of rapid change for midwifery practice and nursing. In Australia these professions are linked by history, education, and regulatory systems. The changes which will affect both groups include the establishment of the Australian Nursing Council (ANC), the acceptance of a university bachelor award as the pre-registration preparation for nurses, and an emerging agreement amongst midwives that they should be university educated. No clear consensus exists, however, about how this should happen.

These developments and debates are occurring within a health system facing economic constraints, and when universities are contracting courses and under pressure to teach more students within current budgets. It is, therefore, necessary to analyse the impact of these issues on a rapidly changing situation in relation to midwifery education.

This analysis is set within the context of increasing opportunities for practice in a range of salaried positions. These include roles in alternative birth centres, in the midwifery teams being established in New South Wales (Rowley 1992, personal communication), which are similar to those reported by Flint et al (1989), and in other initiatives designed to improve women's choices about how they give birth. The conventional hospital services, where the majority of women are still confined, remain the major employers of midwives. Midwives have also greatly increased their involvement in private practice in Australia over the last decade, both conducting home births and confinements in hospitals where they have accreditation. In at least one state, New South Wales, support and policy frameworks are being developed by the Department of Health (New South Wales Department of Health Nursing Branch 1992).

Concurrent with these changes, and not totally unrelated to them, is a rapid reduction in the numbers of obstetricians in training, and an increase in the numbers of obstetricians moving from practices based on normal delivery to 'superspecialisation areas of gynaecology'. This was reported by representatives of the Royal College of Obstetrics and Gynaecology at the 'Birth 2000' meeting, in Sydney, in October 1992.

This chapter explores the context of change and its consequences concerning midwifery education in Australia today. This change will result in preregistration midwifery education being conducted at graduate level within universities in all but one state, should enough places be available, by 1995 (Glover 1992a). The opportunity for education as a midwife in Australia is most likely to remain restricted to registered nurses and to only be available as graduate level study.

## BACKGROUND

### Historical details

Midwifery education in Australia has been undertaken traditionally as a 'second certificate' that followed general nursing. This, in part, reflects our colonisation by Britain and acceptance of a British model of nurse education and practice (Barclay 1985). Variations on this basic model arose, that reflected the geography of Australia and the nature of settlement.

Small cottage hospitals were established that provided all the health needs for an area (Thornton 1972). People would be sent to the city for major surgery but otherwise, between them, the local general practitioner and nurse-midwife would manage the health services for their community. Neither a general nurse without midwifery nor a midwife without nursing skills were employable within cottage hospitals in these circumstances. Home birth became uncommon during the depression for those unable to pay a fee and who could obtain free hospital care.

During the second world war, the nurse-midwives who were not serving with the armed services preferred salaried hospital employment and the emergency back-up services available to them in this role (Thornton 1972).

## Training programs

The educational programs available for students of midwifery varied greatly in organisation, content and hours spent in class-room teaching, between states and territories in Australia, al-though the service employment requirement of 1 year for students remained consistent (Barclay 1985). Barclay's analysis of state and territory requirements for midwifery programs in the early 1980s was repeated by Haddon for the preparation of this chapter, in 1992. Table 6.1 shows that considerable variation persists, with the most comparable aspect being the number of deliveries required of students during their education.

A large and representative study, reported by Barclay in 1984, showed that nearly half of the students on these programs felt inadequately prepared to undertake midwifery practice on grad-uation. Many students were poorly motivated about undertaking the course, and fewer than 60% were employed as midwives within a year of graduating. The excessive wastage rates in graduates reflected the high proportion of students not intending to practise even while they were actually undertaking programs. The study showed antiquated curriculum models; students who claimed they were treated as menial members of the workforce rather than learners; service delivery taking precedence over teaching of students, and students who felt their clinical experi-ence was inadequate for practice (Barclay 1984).

**Table 6.1** Stipulated clinical experience for midwives in Australian states and

| | Labour ward | Outpatients | Postnatal | Antenatal | Nursery | Special care nursery Other | Deliveries |
|---|---|---|---|---|---|---|---|
| NSW[1] | 12 | 2 clinics etc. | | 12 | | 12 | 20 (no more than 5 assisted) |
| VIC[2] | 12 | | 14 | 3 | 12 | 6  1 food-room | 20 (no more than 5 assisted) |
| WA[3] | 10 | | 12 + neonatal ward | 6 | | 8  9 elective clinical experience | 20 (5 may be assisted) |
| QLD[4] | | | | | | | 20 (5 may be assisted) |
| SA[5] | Implementation of individual programmes approved by the NRB and checked annually to ensure they maintain sufficient standard/variety of experience | | | | | | 10 quality |
| ACT[6] | No NRB stipulation but in practice follow the guidelines set down by NSW NRB | | | | | | |
| TAS[7] | Period of time not specified; currently under review. | | | | | | 15 + 5 assists |
| NT[8] | – | 2 | – | – | 8 | 4  –  24 in total | 20 |

[1] New South Wales: NSW Nurses Registration Board (NRB),
[2] Victoria: Midwives Regulations 1985,
[3] Western Australia: Nurses' Regulations 1973,
[4] Queensland: Curriculum Guide Midwifery Nursing Course 1980,

territories. Minimum recommendation in all cases. (Table correct in July 1992)

| Witness | Antenatal examination | Vaginal examination | Complicated pregnancy | Pain management | Episiotomy performance | Observe suturing | Neonatal resuscitation | Tube feeding | Caesarian section | Other |
|---|---|---|---|---|---|---|---|---|---|---|
| 5 before conducting various complicated deliveries | 20 | 10 | 20 | 20 of all types | 2 | 5 | 5 Ob-serve | 5 | 2 | |
| 10 before conducting delivery | | 5 | 5 | 5 inhalational | 3 | | 3 | | 5 | 1 |
| 5 | 5 routine 15 full | 5 | | 5 inhalational; 3 epidural; 2 psycho-prophylaxis | | | | | | |
| 10 before conducting delivery 20 total 10 before conducting delivery | 40 Abdominal | 5 | | 5 inhalational | | | | | 1 | 1 or 2 primi-gravidae in labour |
| 20 | 20 | 10 | | Supervised administration not specified | | | | | | |
| 5 before conducting delivery including: 10 complicated 1 breech 1 forceps 1 caesarian section 1 multiple birth | 15 prenatal 10 abdominal | 14 | | 20 of all types | 2 | 5 | 7 | 5 | 2 | 12 Clinical skills asessments |

[5] South Australia: Currently under review (South Australian Nurses Board),
[6] Australian Capital Territory: Follows NSW (Personal communication, Woden Valley Hospital),
[7] Tasmania: Nusing Board of Tasmania Curriculum Guide,
[8] Northern Territory: Nursing Act Regulations 1983 and Nurses' Registration Board Clinical requirements for midwifery.

## Regulation of midwifery practice in 1984

The regulation of midwifery practice in Australia was also deficient when studied nearly a decade ago. Barclay (1985) argued that this situation had a historic basis from when nursing and medicine combined to regulate and control midwifery. Nursing aligned itself with the medical profession on this issue, because of its concerns to be seen as professionally accountable and to rid itself of the taint of untrained and unregulated practice which was associated with community midwives prepared in apprenticeship systems (Willis 1983). The medical profession, on the other hand, was trying to remove competitors from the field (Forster 1967, Pensabene 1980, Willis 1983). The evidence shows, despite claims by doctors to the contrary, that midwives were operating more safely at this time than their medical counterparts (Lewis 1978).

Regulatory bodies were set up in the states and territories of Australia, by nurses and doctors, to regulate the training and practice of nurses and midwives. This was carried out without ensuring that those structures contained the necessary experience to make judgements on midwifery matters, and without guaranteed midwifery membership (Willis 1983, Barclay 1985). Another important point to consider was that doctors, through their membership of nurses' regulatory boards, were placed in an unique position to protect their own profession's interests and territory in relation to childbirth (Willis 1983).

## CURRENT REGULATIONS GOVERNING THE EDUCATION AND PRACTICE OF MIDWIVES

The author and Haddon undertook to repeat the research reported by Barclay in 1985 for the preparation of this chapter. This involved contacting each state or territory Nurses' Registration Board. The boards were requested to provide all the acts, regulations or guidelines that governed midwifery or midwifery education in that state. It took three telephone calls in most cases to be confident that a full set of these had been obtained; that the data was as accurate as possible, and that documents were not absent. Most states and territories have separate regulations for nurses and midwives. The review showed very little change had occurred in the decade since the previous analysis (Barclay 1985).

This review of regulations governing the registering (licensing) of midwives in Australia shows, as mentioned earlier, that direct

**Table 6.2**  Regulations limiting midwifery to registered general nurses

| States | Regulations |
|---|---|
| New South Wales | Yes. Provision 20, Nurses' Act 1991 |
| Tasmania | No. Nursing Act 1987 |
| Northern Territory | Unclear. Nursing Act 1982 |
| Western Austrlaia | No. Regulation 12(6) Nurses' Regulation 1973 |
| Queensland | Yes. Clauses 158(1) Nursing Bill 1992 allows those previously midwifery-only qualified to continue to be registered. Does not appear to permit new single registered midwives |
| South Australia | Appears to be yes. Registration as a midwife authorises the 'nurse' to practice midwifery, Provision 24(5) Nurses' Act 1984 |
| Victoria | Yes. Regulation 301(a) Midwives' Regulations 1985, Nurses' Act 1985 |
| Australian Capital Territory | Yes. Provision 11(2) Nurses' Act 1988 |

entry midwives are only able to register in a minority of the states of Australia (Table 6.2).

Although most states still do not define midwifery in their documents, the majority now have sufficient guidelines to cover domiciliary practice. There are few stipulations on drug prescription by midwives but most states now provide protocols for emergency care.

Guidelines for antenatal, accouchement, postnatal and infant care have not increased in number. Antenatal care can be provided by midwives independently in only a few states. In Victoria and Tasmania this may only be provided on the authority of a medical practitioner. Whilst all states now have penalties for unregistered practice, these penalties vary from '10 points' in Tasmania[1] to 2 years' imprisonment in the Northern Territory. Although separate guidelines operate for midwives in most states, the term increasingly used in the documents to describe a midwife is midwifery nurse.

---

[1] The documentation provided does not define this penalty further. It is a system only relevant to Tasmania.

## NURSING EDUCATION

The pre-service education of nurses in universities in Australia began in the 1970s. The impetus for this was a concerted push from nursing organisations, and their members, which was maintained over a number of years. This process, not easily achieved and dependent on maintaining a degree of agreement and a unified approach, was well described by Russell (1988). Nurses skilfully combined political process and lobbying with activism, culminating in a march through the city of Adelaide (Garrett 1988). The Commonwealth government committed itself to the transfer of nursing education to the higher education sector in 1984 (Lublin 1985). The maintenance of political pressure has ensured a relatively orderly transition and the provision of university education for all students of nursing in Australia. This transition was completed in 1992.

This is a tremendous achievement and a monument to the nurses' commitment over a 15-year period. Many midwives were involved in this process, if indirectly, because of their dual professional identity as nurses and midwives and as members of nursing and midwifery organisations.

### The transfer of nursing education from hospitals to universities

Nurses did not win every battle in relation to the transfer of nurse education to universities during this period nor were they always united. One area of contention was the duration and nature of the pre-registration award. A number of experienced academics argued that this should be a 4-year degree on the basis that the volume of clinical experience in the program precluded the necessary theoretical content of degree level study. A precedent had been set in Australia, with a number of practice-based professions undertaking 3½- or 4-year degrees, for example nutrition and dietetics, social work and engineering (Universities Admissions Centre (NSW and ACT) 1993). A minority of nursing academics disagree, and supported the notion of a 3-year undergraduate degree in preparation for nursing.

The implementation of a 4-year undergraduate course is obviously more expensive than a 3-year program. As the government underwrites the cost of universities in Australia and students make only a contribution to their education, the government was anxious to ensure a cost-effective transfer of nursing education from hospitals to universities. Previously students had entered 3-year full time diploma programs. Now they enter a degree program of the same duration.

## DIRECT ENTRY TO MIDWIFERY EDUCATION

The opportunity to undertake direct entry midwifery education in Australia has declined, with the disappearance of the last programs about 20 years ago. It must be noted that these programs were only of 1-year's duration, conducted in hospital schools, and whilst they prepared many people who provided valuable and loyal service, would be considered educationally deficient today.

The issue of direct entry to midwifery programs conducted for non-nurses remains contentious in Australia. Strongly held views are expressed by protagonists from both camps. It appears, however, to be an issue for a minority of people rather than one gaining popularity or growing support. For example only two of over 60 midwives who attended a national workshop convened by the Australian College of Midwives Incorporated (ACMI) in Melbourne in March 1992 chose to work on this issue (Glover 1992b, personal communication).

Despite a number of attempts (for example the Direct Entry submission to the Victorian Birthing Services Review, prepared by Shere et al (1989)), neither government nor universities seem to be taking up the challenge of developing such programs. In times of reduced funding available for universities and contraction of the courses being offered, this situation appears unlikely to change.

Graduates of direct entry programs would only be able to register in two of the states of Australia (Table 6.2). This appears to make the re-establishment of direct entry programs even less likely.

## UNIVERSITY AWARDS FOR NURSES AND MIDWIVES

To obtain a degree in nursing a diplomate usually needed to undertake an additional year of full time study. This was usually done following some years of employment as a nurse. Hospital-prepared certificate nurses could also undertake programs of study that prepared them at diploma, or after more extensive study, at degree level. These courses were designed to build on their previous experience in nursing and knowledge, and also provided opportunities for studying social and biophysical sciences frequently missing from the hospital programs. An introduction to nursing science and knowledge was usually a key element of these courses. It was not usual to include clinical experience as students at this stage were experienced nurses.

The first Master of Nursing awards in Australia took graduates with nursing awards together with nurses who had undertaken undergraduate studies in other disciplines (e.g. psychology and education). Again, candidates for these early master's degrees were expert clinicians seeking academic skills for leadership and research (Barclay 1987–1988, unpublished research).

A number of midwives have undertaken these courses and many have been able to undertake research projects into midwifery, supervised by nurse-midwife academics.

Doctoral programs in Australia consist of original research. Candidates will have completed a good undergraduate degree with an additional 'honours' year of research training or a master's degree that contains research. A small number of midwives have completed their doctoral studies. There are a very small number of universities in Australia where supervision of midwife candidates can be undertaken by midwife academics.

## THE AUSTRALIAN COLLEGE OF MIDWIVES (ACMI)

The forerunner of the ACMI was the National Midwives' Association. Formed in 1977 with a membership of a few hundred, the first national conference was held in 1978 in Adelaide (Peters 1991). The Association voted to become autonomous in 1983 and in 1987 constituted the ACMI. The membership is now about 3800 (Higgs 1992, personal communication).

### The role of the ACMI

The ACMI has already provided leadership at a national level in the accreditation of independent or non-salaried midwives. Midwives seeking accreditation complete processes required by the College and any additional steps required by the hospital or health service involved. Unlike Colleges or similar bodies in other countries, the ACMI has not been responsible for examining students or for prescribing experiences required in student programs. Neither has it had a role in monitoring members' credentials, their currency or their credibility.

The resources that the ACMI has available to it, however, are strictly limited as fees for registration to practise, and government support, are channelled into the Nurses' Registration Boards in the various states and territories. It is highly unlikely that this process will change and even more unlikely since the formation of the Australian Nursing Council (ANC). (This issue is discussed more fully later in the chapter.) Unless practising midwives vote to markedly increase their contributions to the ACMI, its role in monitoring the education of midwives or their suitability to practise remains problematic because of lack of resources.

The power bases that have the ear of government on these issues are the nursing organisations to which, paradoxically, many midwives belong because of their dual professional qualifications. The ACMI, however, is the only body with midwifery expertise, and therefore the ANC should refer to it on all midwifery issues. The ACMI has the potential to be a powerful force for ensuring the ANC fulfils its charter in relation to midwifery nursing. If midwifery leadership is ignored at this level, as has occurred over much of this century, an unsatisfactory system will be perpetuated within the new model designed to regulate education and practice in nursing.

## Professional qualifications using the medical model

There is another possibility, at this stage rather remote from achievement, although discussed informally by a number of midwifery leaders: the development of fellowship or similar categories within the college that reflect particular achievement or professional standing. This mechanism could operate along the lines of the well proven medical college model, and the fellowship could become a prerequisite for appointment to particular positions. These positions could include leadership within salaried teams or private practice. Education programs undertaken by candidates, both award and non-award studies, would be one of the aspects scrutinised for fellowship. The clinical experiences of candidates, and their professional standing with colleagues, could be subjected to scrutiny by the college to achieve recognition at the highest level. A similar process is undertaken through the ACMI for accreditation.

Graduates from programs recognised by the ACMI as well as the conferring institution, who have achieved advanced clinical standing and skills, would have a concomitant standing conferred on them within the professional community. Universities seeking recognition for their courses by the ACMI would have to meet criteria determined by the ACMI not just those determined by nurses' boards or the ANC.

*The case against*

Paradoxically though, the achievements already made by nursing and midwifery within the university sector suggest this model may already be superseded. Medicine provides a useful model for comparison. Medical colleges control their own postgraduate education. Candidates within postgraduate medical colleges undertake strictly prescribed clinical and theoretical experiences that are narrowly focused, do not permit more general study, or necessarily challenge professional assumptions about practice. Neither do they permit the attainment of university awards.

Such is the prestige of the medical profession that this is not considered a liability by most, within the profession or by the health system as a whole. It appears, however, to contribute to a professional insularity which makes it difficult for obstetricians to understand changes occurring within Australian society as a whole and within health systems in particular. Obstetricians have little or no exposure to areas of study such as feminism, consumerism and sociology. These are disciplines that help explain the operation of health systems and issues causing major change in health care in midwifery and obstetrics in Australia today.

# A wider approach to professional education

Many midwives lecturing in university-based midwifery courses would claim that one of the major benefits of university education is to move from an instrumental approach to midwifery to a broad theoretical base to practice that does not compromise clinical experience or skill development. Hospital programs achieved high levels of technical proficiency, but universities can offer an education which, without sacrificing competence, enables the graduate to provide leadership and advocacy for women and their families within the professions and community.

Such courses require students to be prepared in political/ professional processes; have available to them sociological and other modes of analysis; be effective health educators and agents and facilitators of change, and be reflective and critical inquirers into their own and others' practice (Barclay 1992). Universities, working alongside expert practitioners who model and teach this approach in practice, can provide the optimal opportunities for this type of education to occur.

## MIDWIFERY EDUCATION IN UNIVERSITIES IN AUSTRALIA

Despite lacking coherent policy direction and agreement about how this should occur, midwifery has moved into universities over the last decade. One of the first courses was at La Trobe University (formerly the Lincoln Institute of Health Sciences) in 1983 (Sledzik 1986). Other universities have been slower to offer midwifery but at the time of writing (1992) there are at least six courses being offered in most Australian states, with a number of new programs planned to commence in 1993.

Midwives, at a meeting associated with the Second National Midwifery Forum in Melbourne in 1991 expressed a strong desire for a uniform approach to this transfer (Sledzik 1992). This call was reiterated at a national meeting convened under the auspices of the ACMI in Melbourne in March 1992. The meeting had as its objective to:

review the provision of midwifery education programs in Australia and to develop a plan for the orderly transfer of midwifery from hospital-based programs to the university sector.

(Glover 1992a)

The rapid pace of change in nursing education has been mirrored in the variety of awards offered over time, and in those that currently prepare aspiring midwives. Midwifery as a pre-service award has been available as a component of a bachelor of nursing degree; as a graduate diploma with or without the option of undertaking further studies to attain a master's degree, and very recently, in two instances only, at master's degree level. There are opportunities for registered midwives to undertake higher degree studies if they have the prerequisite qualifications, but the award is most frequently in nursing.

The variety of awards offered partly reflects the history being created in nursing education in universities but, also, a lack of policy direction and debate about midwifery at national leadership level in professional and educational systems. This debate is now occurring in the midwifery profession. Few people, however, have the necessary experience or influence to ensure the directions taken are coherent and complementary, and that they meet the needs of the community and profession rather than reflect idiosyncratic university or state bias.

Unfortunately the call by the ACMI for an orderly transfer is rather like shutting the stable door after the horse has bolted. What may be more accurately described as a disorderly transfer is well under way. The profession as a whole, or through its organisation (ACMI) is having little impact on universities, who have the power to introduce awards in midwifery that reflect their own academic leadership's view. Diversity of viewpoint and variety of offerings is in fact desirable, but needs to be productive and purposeful and risks lack of coherence and direction at this time.

## Master's degrees and graduate diplomas

One of the major areas of contention is associated with a larger debate within Australian universities about the depth, nature, and duration of master's degrees and the place of graduate diplomas. Graduate diplomas usually build on a relevant undergraduate qualification with 1 year of vocationally focused study. Master's degrees vary within Australian universities, partly depending on whether they are awarded for course work or research or a combination of these. Midwifery awards are considered to be course work degrees, though many programs include preparation in research methods but do no require the student to actually undertake research.

The other complicating factor in this confusing situation is that, in some states, nurses can be admitted to postgraduate study on the basis of prior learning through qualifying studies, without having completed an undergraduate degree. This route of entry is exceptional but ideally suited to nurses who have not had the same access to higher education as other health professions.

The Melbourne meeting reached agreement that the 1-year graduate diploma that follows a nursing qualification is the preferred route for midwifery education (Glover 1992). This was

an important meeting as most university programs were represented.

## Content and title of pre-service courses

Another important debate neither fully explored nor resolved is
the nature of the content in the pre-service award and of its title.
Midwives at the Melbourne meeting, not surprisingly, insisted
that their awards should be described as 'midwifery' rather than
nursing. This debate is not superficial and reflects the deeper issue
that some of these courses are actually embedded within nursing
degrees, while others are more specifically midwifery.

The type of content which can reasonably be seen as inherent
to certain areas of nursing, as well as midwifery, includes topics
such as research methods and family studies. These are content
areas that are also likely to be found in direct entry programs in
other countries. It is the amount of generic nursing content in
relation to specific midwifery content that is contentious and
causing concern in some Australian states and within some
programs.

## THE AUSTRALIAN NURSING COUNCIL

The Australasian Nurse Registering Authorities Conference, the
umbrella meeting of the independent state registering bodies at
which New Zealand is also represented, resolved at its meeting in
Perth in May 1992 that the Australian Nursing Council be
formed. The membership of the Council consists of one representative of each state or territory nurses' board and four
nominated persons, two of whom represent the two major
nursing organisations in Australia. One member represents the
minister responsible for nurse education and one is nominated by
the minister to represent the interests of health consumers
Australian Nursing Council Steering Committee 1992). The powers of this body include:

to co-ordinate all matters relating to the regulation of the nursing
profession in Australia including the education, registration or
enrolment, practice and professional conduct of nurses.

The formation of the ANC is an exciting move towards
rationalising the fragmented regulation of the education and
practice of nurses in Australia. Whether this in any way benefits

midwifery education or practice is problematic. I have argued strongly elsewhere (Barclay 1985) that state nurses' boards were not the optimal bodies to monitor the education and practice of midwives because of their composition and structure. The ANC may well replicate this situation, depending, in part, on the persons nominated to the Council. Without a designated member representing midwives a repeat of the former situation appears highly probable.

The formation of the Australian Nursing Council is a positive step towards professional autonomy for nurses and confirms a hard fought independence from medicine. It perpetuates, however, a view of midwifery as a sphere of nursing practice, which is not necessarily held in the international arena but which is understandable within the Australian historical, geographical and professional context. As previously described, unless the ANC functions with full and appropriate representation, Australian midwives may consider moving outside this system to ensure that their educational and regulatory systems are adequate.

Evidence from research undertaken in the early 1980s suggests both educational and regulatory systems for midwives, controlled by nurses' boards, were seriously flawed (Barclay 1984, 1985). Peters (1991) confirms this position. There is the potential that these flaws will be perpetuated by the ANC.

## CONCLUSION

Australia is a sparsely populated country. It is not possible to determine the exact number of midwives in practice because of dual registration systems of nurses and midwives, and also because the various state and territory nurses' boards have not kept similar databases, allowing meaningful aggregation of the numbers (Peters 1991). The group is small in proportion to the number of registered nurses estimated to be in practice in Australia. Its capacity for generating sufficient revenue to manage its own education and registration affairs is also small.

Despite ideological and professional differences between them, it appears there is no other option but for nurses and midwives to actively collaborate in educational and registration systems. Collaboration will require a greater and more sophisticated involvement of midwives in decision making bodies, with their right of representation as midwives protected. Previous systems have operated poorly in the protection of midwifery standards and in ensuring consistency within educational programs. This situation continues despite evidence from research and strongly expressed concerns by the ACMI. The ANC, established in 1992, has an opportunity to rectify an unsatisfactory situation that has persisted since the early part of the century. It remains to be seen whether this happens.

In the interim, midwifery courses are moving rapidly into universities as postgraduate programs in nursing. The types of courses currently offered vary widely, and new ones do not demonstrate much consistency other than that they generally require 1 year of full time study and clinical experience or equivalent, and are mostly at graduate diploma level. Many courses will permit students who perform well to advance to master's level programs on completion of their course work if they wish. Course brochures demonstrate that these awards are frequently described as awards in nursing or midwifery nursing.

Graduate education for midwives in Australia is a fait accompli. This has resulted from the close links between nurses and midwives. It is also possible for midwives to undertake research degrees within their own area, and increasingly possible to obtain research supervision from midwife researchers who have academic posts at senior levels. These benefits must be balanced by continuing problems of midwife representation on decision making bodies that influence midwives' education and practice. Overall, although the situation remains confused, the achievements of the last decade as nurses and midwives have entered universities have been considerable.

Oakley & Houd (1990) have cautioned midwives on the sociological risks of being professional. In part, their argument is based on the assumption that autonomy is necessary to be professional. However they go on to say that midwives have to follow the directives and leadership of medicine to be identified as professional. In Australia, midwives are less likely at a regulatory level to be dominated by medicine than by nursing. The consequences may be more subtle but are no less real The implications for the education of midwives are profound, particularly at a time of rapid change and transition. Vigilance is necessary to ensure that a system which incorporates both nurses and midwives does so without disadvantaging the smaller group and, by implications, the women and families they serve.

## ACKNOWLEDGEMENT

The research assistance of Yvonne Haddon and the assistance of colleagues who supplied information from a number of areas in Australia are gratefully acknowledged.

REFERENCES

Australian Nursing Council Steering Committee 1992 Establishment of the Australian Nursing Council

Barclay L 1984 An enquiry into midwives' perception of their training. Australian Journal of Advanced Nursing 1(4): 11–24

Barclay L 1985 Australian midwifery training and practice. Midwifery 1: 86–96

Barclay L 1986 One right way: the midwife's dilemma. Unpublished thesis, Canberra College of Advanced Education, Canberra

Barclay L 1987–1988 Unpublished research conducted at Flinders University, South Australia

Barclay L 1992 Education and research: the challenge for midwives of the future. Paper presented at New South Wales Midwives' Association Conference, Penrith, New South Wales, June

Department of Health Nursing Branch 1992 Discussion paper Department of Health of New South Wales

Flint, C, Poulengeris P & Grant A 1989 The 'Know Your Midwife' scheme: a randomised trial of continuity of care by a team of midwives. Midwifery 5(1): 11–16

Forster FMC 1967 Progress in obstetrics and gynaecology in Australia. John Sands, Sydney

Garrett M 1988 Unpublished paper. In part published as: Educating politically aware nurses. Australian Nurses Journal 17(9): 10–11

Glover P 1992a Midwifery education: report of national workshop Australian College of Midwives Journal, June, 5: 7–9

Glover P 1992b Personal communication

Hayes P 1992 Personal communication

Higgs 1992 Personal communication

Lewis M J 1978 Obstetrics education and practice in Sydney, 1870–1939. Australian and New Zealand Journal of Obstetrics and Gynaecology 18:3

Lublin J R 1985 Basic nurse education in CAEs: the educational evidence for transfer. Australian Journal of Advanced Nursing 2(2): 18–28

New South Wales Department of Health Nursing Branch 1992 Discussion paper: nurse practitioners in New South Wales. New South Wales Department of Health, Sydney

Oakley A, Houd S 1990 Helpers in childbirth: midwifery today. Hemisphere, New York

Pensabene T S 1980 The rise and fall of the medical practitioner in Victoria. AMU Press, Canberra

Peters M 1991 Australian midwifery: opportunities and challenges in the next decade. Australian College of Midwives Journal 4(3): 5–10

Rowley M 1992 Personal communication

Russell R L 1988 Nursing education: a time for change 1960–1980. Australian Journal of Advanced Nursing 5(4): 36–44

Shere M, Dempsey R, Deany J, Reynolds K, Chatham E, Fitall A 1989 The journey out: direct entry midwifery. Cited in: Final Report of the Ministerial Review of Birthing Services in Victoria 1990 Having a baby

Sledzik L 1986 Mastery learning for midwifery: a college-based course. Australian Journal of Advanced Nursing 3(2): 46–55

Sledzik L 1992 A conceptual framework for a midwifery curriculum in institutes of higher degree Australian College of Midwives Journal 5(1): 5–9

Thornton A 1972 The past in midwifery services. Australian Nurses' Journal, March, 19–23

Universities Admission Centre (NSW and ACT) 1993 Information guide. Sydney

Willis E 1983 Medical dominance. George Allen & Unwin, Australia

# 7

# The role of graduate education in midwifery in the USA

*Joyce Roberts*

# INTRODUCTION

## Overview of nurse-midwifery education in the US

In 1993 there were 40 nurse-midwifery education programs in the United States that were accredited by the American College of Nurse-Midwives (ACNM) Division of Accreditation (ACNM 1993b). The Division of Accreditation has a major role within the ACNM, establishing the standards for nurse-midwifery education and accrediting education programs (Conway-Welch 1986, Roberts 1991). The current 40 programs include 28 master's-basic education programs, 10 certificate-basic programs, and two pre-certification programs.

The master's-basic programs lead to a master's degree in nursing or public health (MS, MSN, MPH) and eligibility for the national certification examination set by the ACNM Certification Council Inc. (ACC). The certificate-basic programs lead to a certificate in nurse-midwifery post-nursing education and the graduate is also eligible to take the ACC examination. Of the 10 certificate-basic programs, five offer the option of a master's degree through the institution with which they are affiliated. Pre-certification programs are for nurse-midwives who have acquired their midwifery education in another country, or are US-educated nurse-midwives who need to update their knowledge and skills in order to have a current certificate to practice in the US. Upon completion of the pre-certification program, designed for those with previous midwifery education, the individual is eligible for certification in the US (ACNM 1991, Roberts 1991).

All of these nurse-midwifery education programs reside in or are affiliated with an institution of higher education. These include schools of nursing (31), schools of medicine (5), schools of public health (1), or health-related professions (3) (ACNM 1993a). While the programs must be congruent with the graduate program of their institution, the ACNM Division of Accreditation reviews and accredits only the nurse-midwifery curriculum and program.

Graduation from an accredited education program makes an individual eligible to take the national ACNM certification exam. Upon passing this written examination, the graduate is a Certified Nurse-Midwife and may use the initials CNM after his/her name. In 48 states within the US, licensure or authorization to practice as a nurse-midwife requires certification by the American College of Nurse-Midwives. Some states (such as California, Arizona and Washington) also license midwives who complete an education program that is recognized by that state which may not be accredited by the ACNM.

## Focus of this chapter

This chapter will focus on the development of nurse-midwifery education in the United States, extending from initiatives to educate midwives in the early 1900s to the growth of accredited nurse-midwifery programs from 1935 to the present. The formal education of midwives in the United States has been facilitated by their prior education as nurses. The development of financially stable nurse-midwifery education programs has occurred with the placement of midwifery education in post-nursing or post-baccalaureate programs with institutions of higher education. In the post-baccalaureate programs, the student acquires nursing education prior to completing the midwifery education program. Therefore, a certified nurse-midwife (CNM) is a registered nurse with advanced education in midwifery.

Among the current issues in the US regarding the education of the 'professional midwife', are the strategies to educate a greater number of qualified midwives, and the necessity of retaining the nursing prerequisite to formal midwifery education. In 1989 the Carnegie Foundation for the Advancement of Teaching held an invitational meeting with the following goals:

1. better health care for mothers and babies by alleviating the obstetrical care crisis with more midwives, and
2. the promotion of midwifery as a quality profession, requiring emphasis on caring, competence and public education (ACNM 1993a).

As a result of this meeting which included midwives, nurse-midwives and persons from educational institutions and health organizations concerned about these issues, a group of CNMs and other midwives continued to meet as the ACNM/MANA Inter-organizational Workgroup on Midwifery Education. This workgroup included representatives from the American College of Nurse-Midwives (the professional organization of certified nurse-midwives) and the Midwives' Association of North America (MANA), the organization for both empirically and formally educated midwives). This group has continued to debate the definition of the professional midwife, practice competencies and the education of the professional midwife (ACNM 1993a). Addressing the latter issue has included a discussion of the feasibility of educating non-nurses as midwives so as to attain the competencies that have been developed for nurse-midwives. The ACNM is currently exploring how they might expand their criteria in order to accredit a non-nursing-based education program, without altering their established standards for nurse-midwifery education and practice, or jeopardizing the status of the Division of Accreditation as an accrediting agency according to the standards set by the US Department of Education.

In 1982 this Department of the US federal government recognized the ACNM Division of Accreditation as a national accrediting agency (Conway-Welch 1986, ACNM 1991, Roberts 1991). This national recognition enables accredited education programs and their students to be eligible for federal and sometimes non-federal financial assistance. Thus, recognition by the US Department of Education not only reflects the quality of the education standards that have been developed by ACNM through the Division of Accreditation, but also has important funding implications for programs and students. Therefore, the standards of nurse-midwifery education, the financial support of programs and students, as well as philosophical issues related to midwifery education and practice, are all part of the current consideration of whether the established pattern of formal midwifery education in the US should be modified.

This chapter will explore the historical background of these issues. It will describe how midwifery in the United States became so closely associated with nursing and with post-baccalaureate or post-nursing education. The contemporary status of historical issues will be integrated with the chronological discussion of events.

## EARLY HISTORY OF MIDWIFERY IN THE US

### The colonial period

The history of nurse-midwifery in the United States is prefaced by the history of midwifery. Although both nursing and midwifery are traditional roles of women that are inherently linked with the health care of women and children, midwifery predated nursing as we know it today. Modern nursing was not established until 1873, yet there are records of the practice of midwives in the North American colonies in 1630 and of attempts to educate midwives as early as 1762 (Hiestad 1978, Chaney 1980). Midwives were responsible for obstetric care in the colonies for about two and a half centuries (Stern 1972, Roush 1979).

As in Europe at that time, midwifery was outside the realm of legitimate medical practice and was the exclusive preserve of women. Even though professional midwives occasionally arrived in the colonies from Europe, formal midwifery schools were not set up here in this early period of history, despite the efforts of some physicians, like William Shippen Jr in Philadelphia in 1762, to establish schools for midwives. Through the 1800s the native midwife was self- or apprenticeship-taught and was isolated from medicine, nursing or the hospital.

## The 19th century

Increased immigration in the latter part of the 19th century brought more European midwives and physicians, interested in promoting the concept of education for midwifery practice. Free-standing or proprietary schools of midwifery developed in cities such as New York, Philadelphia and Chicago where there were large numbers of foreign-born persons. These programs were viewed as highly inadequate (Litoff 1978, DeVitt 1979). However, the midwives trained in European schools of midwifery were viewed as having 'far more rigorous obstetric training than nearly all the medical schools in the United States' (DeVitt 1979).

The decline and disappearance of US midwifery schools is attributed to financial instability; limited clinical experience; criticism of the lack of a sound theoretical base, and the decline in the immigration rates of populations who preferred midwifery services. In addition, social, feminist and philosophical issues were involved in this decline.

Although some historians attribute the elimination of the midwife primarily to the development of professional obstetrics within the practice of medicine (Litoff 1978, 1982), Hiestad (1978) concluded that the lack of formal education programs, and 'the failure to maintain rigorous requirements for midwives, for the most part, caused the demise of [midwifery's] occupational identity'. DeVitt (1979) as well as Litoff (1982) identified the lack of professional organization accompanying the midwives' ethnic and racial minority status as key factors contributing to the suppression of the midwife in America. Stern (1972) summarized the variety of social, economic and health care patterns that were related to the decline in midwifery practice as follows:

By the end of the nineteenth century, a series of social and economic events occurred which resulted in the decline of the native midwife. Between 1900 and 1935, her share of deliveries had fallen from about 50 to 10%. Her clientele of foreign-born in the cities was becoming integrated, and new immigration laws prevented their replacement. Home deliveries were being replaced by those in the hospital at which the native midwife had no privileges. The urban indigent were beginning to receive prenatal care at the maternity clinics of large city hospitals. It was a new scientific age; the public was becoming affluent, and attitudes toward childbearing were changing. Pregnancy and delivery could be a hazardous process, but the new obstetrician instead of nature would be responsible for a safe and happy outcome. Physicians had become increasingly critical of the midwife.

Exceptions to this pattern in America existed in a unique social context, that of the Mormon pioneer midwives. Cameron (1967) described their history from 1812 through 1932. The Mormons initially relied on midwives who had been trained in their native lands, and then made deliberate efforts to access the medical-obstetrical education that was available at that time. Those Mormon women who could travel to the East to study at the Women's Medical College in Philadelphia, in 1874 and during the following few years, brought back their knowledge and established midwifery courses in the state of Utah to which they had migrated. From 1894, when licensure for practice was required, through 1932 when the last license was issued, 208 midwives were licensed in Salt Lake. Along with an incentive to acquire midwifery training, these women lived in a part of the United States which, at that time, was very remote and where competition with physicians was not a deterrent to the education of midwives nor to their practice.

## MIDWIFERY IN THE 20TH CENTURY

Although the quality of medical obstetrical care at the start of the 20th century was no better than midwifery care, there were major reforms of medical education subsequent to the Flexner Report of 1910. There was no similar avenue to improve the education or preparation of the midwife. Not only were there no recognized midwifery schools, women were not permitted to enrol in the medical schools that were being established. Since there were few opportunities available to midwives for obtaining new knowledge, the quality of midwifery practice gradually fell behind that of the medical man of that time. Without opportunity for training or supervision, much of midwifery fell into the hands of women who were frequently superstitious and ignorant (van Blarcom 1911, 1914).

In addition to the lack of educational opportunities, the underlying attitude of midwives toward childbirth as 'normal' and inherently within the female domain of competence may also have prevented them from seeking formal education. Wertz & Wertz (1990) proposed that:

Doctors were unable to attract women for training [as midwives], perhaps because women were uninterested in studying what they thought they already knew and, moreover, studying it under the tutelage of men.

They concluded that:

the restraints of traditional modesty and the tradition of female sufficiency for the management of birth were apparently stronger than the appeal of a rationalized system for a more scientific and, presumably, safer midwifery system.

Male attitudes towards women also contributed to doctors' opposition to midwives. Some male physicians contended that 'women were unsafe to attend deliveries and that no "true" woman would want to gain the knowledge and skills necessary to do so' (Wertz & Wertz 1990). Thus, sexist attitudes as well as the midwives' inherent beliefs about childbirth converged to discourage formal education.

Therefore, the perspective of the midwife concerning childbirth and formal education, the social bias against women, along with attitudes about their proper role in society, contributed to their exclusion from medical schools.

In addition, as the physicians became more educated, childbirth became viewed less as a normal process and more as a potentially abnormal event. The physician became more reliant on intervention during pregnancy and childbirth and less reliant, as was the midwife, on nature. In contrast to the European pattern of medical and midwifery education, where doctors were often trained in normal obstetrics by midwives, the two practitioners in the United States were not educated together and came to represent two distinctly different philosophies of birth.

Some early influential obstetricians actively promoted the philosophy that birth was 'pathologic', in order to exclude the midwife who was not prepared to deal with events outside the 'natural'. One of these obstetricians was DeLee who in 1915 wrote:

Obstetrics has a great pathologic dignity – it is a major science of the same rank as surgery . . . even natural deliveries damage both mothers and babies, often and much. If childbearing is destructive, it is pathogenic, and it if is pathogenic it is pathologic . . . If the profession would realize that parturition viewed with modern eyes is no longer a normal function, but that it has imposing pathologic dignity, the midwife would be impossible even of mention

(DeLee 1915 in DeVitt 1982)

Thus, a philosophical schism was exposed that began to influence the societal perception of childbirth as well as putting the midwife at odds with the obstetrician. These philosophical issues persist. At that time they began to influence women's concerns the expectations regarding maternity care as childbirth became 'medicalized' (Dye 1986, Eakin 1986).

American women, especially those of the middle and upper class, came to prefer, and in fact seek out, the promise of safety in childbirth along with more respectability (Dye 1986, Eakin 1986, Wertz & Wertz 1990). Thus, changing population patterns limited the practice of indigenous midwives to the urban or rural ethnic minorities or poor, while social attitudes limited the education of women as midwives and also endorsed the care of women during childbirth by men.

## The 'midwife problem'

Despite the increased involvement of physicians in maternity care and the movement of birth from the home into the hospital, the rate of infant and maternal mortality in the United States in the early 1900s remained alarmingly high. In addition, the high incidence of infant blindness contributed to the controversy known as the 'midwife problem'. Continued practice by midwives was cited as the cause for poor birth outcomes and their unhygienic care as the source of infant blindness (Kobrin 1966). Their immigrant status, ignorance, lack of training and unsupervised practice were the basic underlying causes of the poor quality of care associated with midwives (Abbott 1915).

However, it was learned that the practice of obstetrics was less than exemplary (Kobrin 1966). In 1912 a survey was carried out by J. Whitridge Williams, an esteemed Professor of Obstetrics at Johns Hopkins University in Baltimore, Maryland. Williams (1912) found that:

the average practitioner, through his lack of preparation for the practice of obstetrics, may do his patients as much harm as the much-maligned midwife.

With a high degree of candor he reported further that:

more deaths occur each year from operations improperly performed by practitioners than from infections in the hands of midwives.

Similarly, a 1914 report by Carolyn van Blarcom, the RN appointed to the New York Committee for the Prevention of Blindness, stated:

However, bad the midwife is, we are sorry to have to admit that on the whole a patient is often better off in her hands than in the care of many of the physicians who compete with her. Investigations which have been made concerning the etiology of ophthalmia neonatorum and puerperal septicemia indicate that more of these cases are to be traced to physicians than to midwives.

Miss van Blarcom thought that it was bad enough that:

The desire of foreign women to employ midwives and the determination of midwives to be employed is so strong that even were midwives legislated out of existence they would still be called in by expectant mothers who instead of paying the fee as such, would leave the usual sum of $5 or $10 in some place where the midwives would be sure to see it.

but worse,

if midwives were eliminated many of the patients now being attended by them would fall into the hands of that class of practicing physicians which at present is doing as much or even more actual harm than the midwives themselves.

Carolyn van Blarcom concluded further,

It would appear that the only course for general adoption toward the solution of this problem in America would be the training, licensure and control of midwives where ever they are practicing to any great extent.

She, herself, participated in the establishment of the Bellevue School for Midwives and became known as 'the first nurse in the United States to be licensed as a midwife' (Hawkins 1987). In contrast, Williams recommended the abolition of midwives along with better education of physicians.

## Birth outcomes

As the midwifery debate continued, the number of midwives as well as the deliveries by them decreased. However, the overall health statistics representing the wellbeing of mothers and infants did not improve. It is ironic that the negative indicators actually rose as the practice of midwives declined (DeVitt 1979). It is also ironic, but reflective of the other powerful social and physician influences, that the practice of midwives declined despite evidence of the lower maternal and infant mortality rates that were achieved by them. These lower rates were reported for sectors of the eastern cities of Newark, New Jersey (Levy 1918) and New York (Baker 1913), where services by midwives were retained, and assessed by comparison to the rates for other services or cities.

The better outcomes associated with midwifery deliveries are even more remarkable if one considers that the midwives were primarily attending births in very poor and disadvantaged families. Then, as now, infant mortality was highly correlated with the father's/family's income which was related to living conditions and access to adequate services, food, water and housing. It would have been more likely for the women cared for by midwives to have had poorer outcomes, for these socioeconomic reasons (DeVitt 1979). The poorer birth outcomes for physicians was attributed to their use of measures to hasten labor which were not used by midwives, as well as to the physicians' lack of training and experience with childbirth (Litoff 1978, DeVitt 1979, Bogden 1986).

These favorable midwifery outcomes would be noted, however, along with the successes achieved by midwives in Germany (Emmons & Huntington 1912, Hardin 1925) and England (Noyes 1912), by physician and nursing leaders who believed that trained midwives could and should play a role in the provision of maternity care. The outcome would be the integration of the role of the midwife and the public health nurse in the individual prepared as a nurse-midwife.

## Interfacing of nursing and midwifery

Subsequent reviews of this 'problem' advocated (in addition to improved standards of medical education and obstetrical practice) the involvement of midwives supervised by nurses (Ziegler 1922). This strategy of interfacing nursing and midwifery was advocated by both nursing and physician writers, who saw the extension of nursing responsibility as a way to influence the quality of maternity care by midwives. Nursing leaders, such as Carolyn van

Blarcom (1914) advocated the use of nurses trained as midwives as a solution to some of the most critical aspects of childbirth care, specifically the use of aseptic and hygienic practices that would reduce the incidence of infant blindness. A physician, Herbert Stowe, at Chicago Lying-In Hospital also advocated the specialized training of the nurse in obstetrics (Stowe 1910). He did not call this nurse a midwife, but rather a 'specially trained obstetric nurse' whose responsibility would 'correspond with ... the obstetric specialist. The work of the two go hand in hand' (Stowe 1910).

These perspectives were controversial, and at this point some consideration of the education and role of nurses is required.

## Nursing and midwifery

During the early 1900s nursing education became established in the United States. Although Florence Nightingale (1871) considered midwifery to be 'another branch of nursing art' (van Blarcom 1911), requiring the training of women for services among the poor, early American nursing leaders did not consider midwifery to be part of nursing preparation or practice. In 1901 when Lavina Dock (Robb et al 1901) reported on nursing education in the United States, she included obstetrics as part of the generally accepted course of study. Dock pointed out, however, that:

The nurse never takes up midwifery work, and in private practice or district nursing goes only to obstetric cases where a doctor is in attendance ... The midwife question, so distracting in other countries, does not exist here as a complication to nurses, and is consequently a question that we may leave to the medical profession to settle.

Not only did these nursing leaders not view midwifery as an extension of nursing, in the early decades of the 20th century it was also difficult to train nurses in obstetric care because the majority of births at that time were in the home, not in the hospitals where the nursing schools were being established. Maternity care was largely carried out within the community. Therefore, the nurses who were involved with the 'supervision of midwives' were primarily involved in public health and community nursing.

There were several nurses who were concerned about maternal and child health care and who were actively involved in social and health reforms. One of these nurses was Lillian Wald who in 1903 founded the New York Henry Street Settlement and also suggested a federal Children's Bureau. This unit of the federal government, established between 1909 and 1912, played a major role in health reforms, and subsequent midwifery practice, by promoting birth and death registration and investigating matters related to the health care of children. Their studies made it apparent that infant health is inseparable from maternal health and the quality of maternity care. Other studies confirmed that early and continuous prenatal care could help prevent both maternal and infant deaths. The initiatives supported by the Children's Bureau called for public health nurses to provide prenatal instruction and services.

The role of the nurse was augmented by another key item of federal legislation, the Sheppard–Towner Act of 1921, which provided grants to states for the training of native midwives by public health nurses. Ironically, as legislation in many of the states between 1900 and 1930 was attempting to regulate the midwife out of existence, federal legislation was expanding the responsibility of nurses in the provision of maternity services and for the supervision of the indigenous midwives that still practised. Thus, nurses in public health became more and more involved in maternity care.

## Politics and public health

The political aspect of these legislative initiatives related to social and health care reform should also be acknowledged. Tom (1982) noted that during World War I the limited fitness of men for military service was recognized. A third of the men examined for the military were deemed to be physically unfit for service (Parsons 1921). This finding caused physicians and public health officials to realize that: 'something must be done to remedy the conditions which made such a thing possible in America in the twentieth century' (Parnall 1921, cited by Tom 1982). Not only was a large proportion of men unqualified, but it was determined that, probably one-half of these young men could have qualified for the fighting line if they had been properly cared for during childhood' (Parsons 1921, cited by Tom 1982). Thus, the focus sharpened on maternal and child health care, as Parnall (1921, cited by Tom 1982) asserted:

No community can afford not to assure its future citizens the right to be well born. That is, to be born sound and to live and develop into usefulness . . . The mother who at times, in imminent risk of her own life, furnishes the State with its greatest asset, is entitled to every possible consideration. Proper maternity care should be her right

Tom (1982) goes on to state:

It is important to note that the outpouring of state and federal funds into public health programs was not promoted by the appallingly high maternal and infant mortality rates in the United States. Even though World War I was justified as 'the war to end all wars', the government was insuring itself for future wars by ploughing money into public health. For the first time children were recognized at future members of the military and thus deserving of federal funds. Similarly, women were recognized as producers of future fighting men, and their health became a national resource.

The most visible result of these insights and the concern for maternal and child health was the Sheppard–Towner Act of 1921, mentioned above, which expanded the role of public health nurses in maternity care and in the supervision of indigenous midwives. The administering federal agency was the Children's Bureau.

Despite the national need for improved maternity services, the Sheppard–Towner Act was a controversial bill in the national Congress of the United States. Opponents tried to defeat it by calling it 'federal midwifery'. Nevertheless, the Bill passed as the result of one of the most effective expressions of women's political influence (Chafe 1972). The Sheppard–Towner Act was allowed to lapse in 1929 due to opposition by the American Medical Association (AMA). The AMA opinion reflected the opposition of physicians to midwives because of their desire to establish a 'single standard' of obstetrical care, and also because they realized that the expansion and licensing of midwivery would mean governmental regulation of their own practice also (DeVitt 1979).

## THE EMERGENCE OF THE NURSE-MIDWIFE

### Role differentiation: nurse/midwife and nurse-midwife

There continued to be a need for improved maternity services, opposition to midwives by physicians, and controversy in nursing about the role of nurses in the practice of obstetrics.

In 1909 the American Society of Superintendents of Training

Schools for Nurses (ASSTSN) directed that nurses' training in obstetrics should be limited to emergencies, to observing symptoms and reporting problems, or to a broad general preparation. 'Good obstetric nursing' included such activities as bathing the mother and child, making the bed, and looking after the patient's general comfort (ASSTSN 1909). In 1911 the Society passed a resolution to work toward provision, 'for suitable training, registration, licensure, supervision and control of women engaged in the practice of midwifery' (ASSTSN 1911).

That same year, the Bellevue School for Midwives in New York City began to educate midwives. Its opening was a result of the efforts of Carolyn van Blarcom, the nurse mentioned earlier, who advocated the practice of midwifery in her efforts to improve health care for mothers and infants, specifically to prevent infant blindness. Another nurse, Clara Noyes, who was Superintendent of Training Schools, Bellevue and Allied Hospitals, including the School for Midwives, also supported the education of nurses as midwives. In an address before the International Congress of Hygiene and Demography in 1912 she said,

It is not improbable to expect that advanced obstetrical training will eventually be given to nurses in this country to fit them to carry their share of this problem of mothers and babies. If the midwife can gradually be replaced by the nurse who has, upon her general training superimposed a course in practical midwifery, which has been clearly defined by obstetricians, it would seem a logical solution to the problem . . . We should be able to provide better teaching, better nursing, and eventually better medical assistance to the less highly favored classes.

The midwifery program at Bellevue was supported by public taxes from 1911 until 1935 when the city's 'diminishing need for midwives no longer justified its existence' (Speert 1980). Hemschemeyer (1939) indicated that the closure of this school 'was no reflection on the midwives' work nor on the school, for coincident with the decrease in this midwife group was a similar increase in hospital facilities for maternity care'. The practice of midwifery was limited to home births, and with the movement of childbirth to the hospital, the midwife was excluded.

Following the successful introduction of general public health nurses into maternity centers in the 1920s and early 1930s, a collaborative proposal to educate nurse-midwives, by the Maternity Center Association in New York and the Bellevue School of

Midwifery, was opposed by various medical and nursing leaders (Hiestad 1978). Thus, nurses, in general, did not aspire to practice midwifery, physicians viewed childbirth as a medical responsibility to be undertaken in the hospital setting, and the practice of midwives diminished. In New York City in 1919, 30% of live births were attended by midwives; by 1929, 12%; and by 1939, 2% (Hemschemeyer 1939).

## Nurses educated to supervise midwives

The need remained for improved maternal/child health services and the practice of midwives continued. This need led to advanced preparation of public health nurses to supervise midwives' practice and eventually to the preparation of nurses as nurse-midwives. The latter grew out of the involvement of public health nurses in midwifery practice, as authorized by the Sheppard–Towner Act. In overseeing the practice of 'lay' midwives, the public health nurses provided direction in aseptic practice and maternal and child care and hygiene, but they did not know midwifery practice. The public health nurses were restricted in their ability to train and 'supervise' practising midwives because of the limited attention to maternity care within nursing education. Besides this, there was increased recognition that the real solution to the 'midwife problem' was not the supervision of midwives, but rather their education, as expressed by Carolyn van Blarcom (1914):

Registration, supervision and control are important only as secondary measures, for the foundation upon which all of this work must inevitably rest is through preparatory training.

Thus, there continued to be an expression of the need for midwifery services by trained midwives.

According to Shoemaker (1947), the 'very first school for nurse-midwifery to be established in the United States, although it was not officially recognized, was the Manhattan Midwifery School founded in 1928 in connection with the Manhattan Maternity and Dispensary in New York'. Shoemaker's 1947 historical dissertation on nurse-midwifery in the United States reported what little could be found out about this short-lived school. It was started by a public health nursing instructor from a district nursing association, Mary Richardson, who had taken a midwifery course in England. Although it is not clear what happened to this school, two of its graduates were identified as joining the Frontier Nursing Service in 1928 (the *Quarterly Bulletin of the Frontier Nursing Service*, IV(2):12, in Schoemaker (1947)). Shoemaker's brief account reflects the pattern of development of nurse-midwifery education in the US, which involved the initiative of nurses to educate public health nurses as midwives, based on the British model of nurse-midwifery education.

Also numbered among the public health nurses who were addressing the need for maternity services was Hattie Hemschem-eyer, a future nurse-midwife and first president of the American College of Nurse-Midwives. She observed:

The bulk of nursing care of mothers confined at home is not being done by the professional nurse . . . Nursing in the United States has never developed a clear attitude toward the professional responsibilities which might be considered as minimum essentials for the care of every patient, nor has it gone out and crusaded on a broad front for help to do this task. I do not mean to belittle the efforts made by the (nursing) profession, but it is clear to all who study that the European system assures every mother of some nursing care given by the trained midwife.

Thus, from an historical perspective, nurse-midwifery in the United States can be characterized by the preparation of nurses with public health nursing experience as midwives. The initial nurse-midwifery services and education programs at the Frontier Nursing Service in Kentucky in 1925 (service) and the Maternity Center Association in New York City in 1932 (education) were public health-oriented, as were other nurse-midwifery services which developed, such as that in Santa Fé, New Mexico in 1943.

## First recognized nurse-midwifery school

In New York in 1931 the Lobenstine Midwifery Clinic was established, for teaching midwifery to public health nurses so that they could supervise immigrant and rural midwives still in practice (Maternity Center Association 1943). This initiative became the earliest midwifery education program for nurses. The School of the Association for the Promotion and Standardization of Midwifery, opened in 1932. In the selection of the first class of students, priority was given to nurses from states that had high infant mortality rates and many lay midwives. It was expected that the graduates would return to their home states and establish public health department programs for training and supervising 'granny midwives' (Hogan 1975).

The School was merged with the Lobenstine Clinic under the Maternity Center Association (MCA) in 1934, and thereafter was known by the name of that Clinic. Hattie Hemschemeyer, a public health nurse educator was a graduate of its first nurse-midwifery class and was appointed as Director. Along with preparation to supervise lay midwives, there was an emphasis on the provision of care to women during pregnancy and childbirth, through neighborhood clinics staffed by public health nurses and physicians. The prototype of this type of service was the Maternity Center Association in New York, established in 1918, which developed approximately 30 centers in New York City. Nurse-midwifery services were initiated by the MCA in 1931 and through these centers the role of the nurse-midwife was developed in a way that involved close medical supervision (Hemschemeyer 1939, Walsh 1991). Thus, the role of the public health nurse evolved into that of the nurse-midwife.

## Continued role differentiation: obstetric nurse or nurse-midwife

The role of the nurse in maternity care was also developing and was differentiated from midwifery and medical practice. The Preston Retreat School of Midwifery, is mentioned in historical accounts as a maternity hospital for 'indigent married women' and school for midwives that was operated by two nurse-midwives in 1923 in Philadelphia. It apparently converted to the training of graduate nurses due to 'the diminished need for native midwives in that city' (Shoemaker 1947).

However, the role of the nurse was not that of midwife. Reports from the National League of Nursing Education around that time described the role of the nurse in obstetrics as related more to the overall promotion of the health and comfort of the mother and baby, which supplemented the role of the physician (National League for Nursing Education 1937). According to Hall (1927), the obstetric nurse was a 'bedside assistant' and 'teacher of health'. Henderson stated that:

obstetrical nursing is chiefly a matter of health guidance for the mother, assistance to the mother during and immediately following delivery and hygienic care of the infant.

(Harmer & Henderson 1955)

Thus, as in the earliest decades of the 20th century, the nurse felt, and indeed was, generally unprepared in obstetrics (Corbin 1946, Keane 1959).

Along with the development of programs in nurse-midwifery, advanced courses in maternity nursing also were offered during the 1940s, in order to improve the education of nurses in maternity care. Some of these 'postgraduate' courses reflected a concept of midwifery as well as advanced maternity nursing. However, the emphasis in nursing became more oriented towards a supportive and educative role (Roberts 1984), while nurse-midwifery education included these dimensions of maternity nursing along with midwifery practice and preparation to become supervisors, teachers and consultants in maternity care (Walsh 1991).

Midwifery was viewed by nurses as 'medical practice' (Reinders, cited in Tom 1982) and it would not be until the later part of the 20th century (1968) that organized nursing regcognized the nurse-midwife as a specialty within nursing (American Nurses' Association 1968).

Nurse-midwives have recently been described by nursing leaders as 'the oldest of the specialized practice roles for nurses' and as providing 'an unusually good example of the issues nursing faces in addressing public policy considerations of manpower, economics, costs of care, quality and access to care, and interprofessional politics' (Diers 1982). The nurse historian Hiestad concluded her 1978 review of nurse-midwifery education in the United States by saying, 'Nurse-midwives have served us well. Their mature, intelligent dedication to the public and to their profession makes this one of the proudest chapters in nursing history' (Hiestad 1978). Despite this recognition, nurse-midwives continue to address the issue of their relationship with nursing as well as with 'lay' midwives (Lubic 1982, Sharp 1983, ACNM 1993a).

## Nurse? Midwife? Obstetrical assistant? Nurse-midwife!

It should be noted that just as nurses were initially mixed in their opinions about the role of nurses in midwifery practice, the earliest nurse-midwives were reluctant to be identified as midwives 'because of the prejudice it [the title midwife] arouses'

(Hemschemeyer 1939). Hattie Hemschemeyer, one of the first American nurse-midwives, mixed the terms 'obstetrical nurse' and 'nurse-midwife'. In describing midwifery and the education of nurse-midwives in the United States, she said (1939):

These women, for the time being, are called nurse-midwives. One of their greatest handicaps is their title. There is no point in making any bones about it; to some people the very work is like a red rag to a bull. Nurse-midwives need another name which describes their functions more acceptably to the public as well as to the profession and which leaves the person who uses the title, or who hears it used, free from prejudice.

Some graduates of the early nurse-midwifery education programs 'tucked away the title of midwife' (Hemschemeyer 1939) because it was a handicap in their positions. The earliest physician advocates of nurse-midwives recommended the title 'obstetrical assistant' (Eastman 1953, 1962) because 'to the vast majority of obstetricians the very word midwife is anathema, whether or not it is coupled with the term nurse' (Eastman 1962), and 'because it ['obstetrical assistant'] more nearly connotes than any other the main function which we would envisage for such nurses, namely, the rendering of skilled assistance to obstetricians' (Eastman 1953).

This differential response to titles was evident in the first survey of physician attitudes towards nurse-midwifery, carried out by the Children's Bureau in 1962 (Thomas 1965). The survey was sent to the membership of the American College of Obstetricians and Gyneocologists (ACOG). Approximately 50% of the fellowship responded with replies from 3307 physicians. In the questionnaire where the term 'nurse-midwife' was used there was 'a very low favorable response'. When the functions of a nurse-midwife were attributed to a person called 'a well-trained graduate maternity nurse' the items 'received an amazingly high favorable response' (Thomas 1965).

Despite this perspective of physicians, nurse-midwives were clear in their purpose:

to provide the best possible nursing care for families having a baby ... and not as a stop-gap emergency worker filling a void left by unavailable personnel, nor is she an obstetric technician, extending the hands and feet of the busy physicians.

(Keane 1965 p 2)

They were also highly committed to professional nursing, to

which they had 'added the knowledge and skills of midwifery, in order to be able to do what was already being required of nurses who were 'empirically practicing some aspect of midwifery every day' (Keane 1965). Keane (1965) maintained that:

Nurse-midwifery practice is nothing 'new' on the American nursing scene. It is only its formalization as a professional discipline that makes it seem new!

Both nurse-midwives and physicians found their identity as highly skilled nurses more acceptable.

Therefore, nurse-midwives' identity and education as nurses was a critical aspect in their acceptance within the US health care system. In addition, the extension of the education of public health nurses initially with the intent to 'supervise the untrained midwives . . . and also, under the direction of obstetricians, bring skilled care to the mothers in isolated rural areas' (Maternity Centre Association 1943) was the most viable means to educate midwives and address the societal needs for quality maternity care. Although the early nurse-midwives were adamant about retaining the title of nurse-midwife (because 'it identified them with their colleagues in Europe and elsewhere, where nurse-midwife is an accepted and respected title' (Corbin & Hellman 1960), it would not be until the late 1960s and early 1970s that the title 'Certified Nurse-Midwife' was used openly with pride and a sense of competence and status in the provision of nurse-midwifery care.

The early nurse-midwives recognized, as do contemporary ones (Varney 1987), that nursing and midwifery are two distinct professions (Hemschemeyer 1957). However, they recognized that, 'Midwifery will develop [in the US] only as it is combined with professional nursing under medical direction' (Hemschemeyer 1957). Thus, the social context for nurse-midwifery education and practice was still hostile towards midwifery as the initial schools developed.

However, the need for midwifery services persisted, and committed and courageous individuals from both nursing and medicine continued to advocate quality maternity care through the utilization of nurse-midwives. These factors of need for maternity services and social/professional acceptability, together with the post-basic nature of midwifery education as an advanced nursing specialty, requiring leadership and educational capabilities as well as practice skills, influenced the placement of nurse-midwifery education within institutions of higher education.

## Affiliation with academic institutions and hospitals

A unique and crucial aspect of the initial nurse-midwifery education program was its association with an institution of higher education, Teachers' College, Columbia University, in New York. This assured a sound theoretical base in public health nursing (Hemschemeyer 1932, 1939). Another unique feature of this initial education program was the absence of a hospital affiliation. It would be another 21 years before the graduates were allowed to enter a hospital, and even then it was to establish parent education programs. In 1955 Columbia–Presbyterian–Sloane Hospital in New York City became the first institution of organized medical care to open its doors to nurse-midwives (ACNM 1958, Roush 1979). From there, the provision of nurse-midwifery services, including the conduct of deliveries, spread.

Between 1933 and 1953, most of the 231 MCA graduates worked in public health agencies of public clinics, not in private midwifery practice. Although there were conspicuous efforts not to compete with physicians for patients, and to emphasize the supervisory role of the obstetrician, nurse-midwives became more involved in the provision of direct maternity services (Hemschemeyer 1939, Eastman 1958). Over a 26-year period the Maternity Center Clinic nurse-midwives attended over 6000 births, and reported a maternal mortality rate of 0.9 per 1000 live births at a time when the national average was 10.4 per 1000. In 1958 the Maternity Center School of Nurse-Midwifery moved to the State University of New York in Brooklyn and developed a nurse-midwifery clinical practice at Kings County Hospital (Walsh 1991).

Thus, nurse-midwifery education became more oriented to the preparation of nurse-midwives for the provision of clinical services, instead of for supervisory roles, and the education program retained in association with an established institution of higher education. The experience of these nurses in public health led them to develop nurse-midwifery practices that were characterized by family-oriented health care, an awareness of cultural and environmental factors, and a multidisciplinary approach (Walsh 1991).

# THE DEVELOPMENT OF NURSE-MIDWIFERY SERVICES

## The Frontier Nursing Service

Although the Maternity Center Association was the first organization to plan the education of the nurse-midwife and her introduction into public maternity services, the MCA Nurse-Midwifery Service initiated in 1931 was the second American service of its kind. The Frontier Nursing Service was the first organization to implement nurse-midwifery as an integral aspect of a rural public health services (Breckenridge 1952).

In 1925 the Frontier Nursing Service began offering care to mothers and families in the rugged Kentucky mountains under the leadership of Mary Breckenridge. She chose this remote rural setting to demonstrate the efficacy of nurse-midwifery as a system of maternity and infant care (Dye 1983). Public health nurses, trained in Britain as midwives, provided services in districts surrounding a central hospital in Hyden, Kentucky. This service still holds as a model of planning and providing essential health care, with midwifery care as a major dimension. Nevertheless Dye (1983) views this nurse-midwifery model and the Frontier Nursing Service as 'an anomaly in the American health care system', because of their emphasis on normality in a social context of increasing reliance on operative intervention, hospitalization and the medical management of maternity care.

It was no 'accident' that this model service was characterized as a nursing service, or that the midwives who practised, and subsequently, those who were educated, within it were and are nurse-midwives. Mary Breckenridge very systematically assessed first the health care needs of the population in that region of the country, and then how similar needs were addressed in other countries. She traveled to France (where midwives were not nurses) and England (where midwives were also nurses) and concluded that 'nurse-midwifery was the logical response to the needs of the young child in rural America' (Breckenridge M 1952). She saw midwifery services within the broad context of health care that needed to be provided in Hyden, Kentucky, as well as in other urban or rural areas, and decided that the midwife needed a broad background in nursing practice as well as midwifery. Thus, the initial nurse-midwifery education program as well as the initial service were based on the British model of a nurse educated also as a midwife (ACNM 1958).

When the supply of British-trained nurse-midwives was diminished because of World War II, an education program, the second in the United States, was developed at the Frontier Nursing Service for nurses. The Maternity Center Association in New York assisted with this effort. Again, as with World War I, an international war effort impacted on the education of nurse-midwives.

The publicity given to the work of the Frontier Nursing Service brought the concept of the nurse-midwife to the attention of the public. This publicity came not from the nurse-midwives themselves, but from a report of a major life insurance company, Metropolitan Life, which studied the first 1000 deliveries. Dr Louis Dublin, third Vice President and statistician wrote:

> The most important single result of this work is that not one of the women died as the direct result of either pregnancy or labor . . . The study shows conclusively what has in fact been demonstrated before, that the type of service rendered by the Frontier Nurses safeguards the life of mother and babe. If such service were available to the women of the country generally, there would be a saving of 10 000 mothers' lives a year in the United States, there would be 30 000 less stillbirths and 30 000 more children alive at the end of the first month of life.
>
> (Willeford 1933)

It is ironic that an impetus to the expansion of nurse-midwifery services in our earliest history and at the present was and is influenced by insurance companies. In a contemporary context, health insurers are viewing nurse-midwives favorably because of their cost-effectiveness (Reid & Morris 1979, Diers 1982, Rooks 1990). This recognition, and subsequent repeated documentation, of the positive contributions of nurse-midwives exacerbated what has become an ongoing problem: that of educating a sufficient number of nurse-midwives. Thus, despite the 'anomalous' nature of nurse-midwifery, the need for maternity services and the recognition of the quality and 'cost-effectiveness' of nurse-midwifery services have contributed to the increased acceptance of their practice and current demand for nurse-midwives.

As the percentages in Table 7.1 indicate, there have been increased opportunities for nurse-midwives to practise. Although these percentages are still disproportionately small, especially when compared to midwifery practice in other countries, they are a reflection of the recognition of the quality of certified nurse-

**Table 7.1** Nurse-midwives in clinical practice[1] and US births delivered by midwives.[2] CNM, certified nurse-midwife.

| Year | Percentage of CNMs in practice | Year | Percentage of births delivered by midwives |
|------|-------------------------------|------|-------------------------------------------|
| 1963 | 11 | | |
| 1967 | 23 | | |
| 1971 | 37 | | |
| | | 1975 | 0.9 |
| 1976 | 50 | | |
| 1982 | 66 | 1982 | 1.8 |
| 1987 | 70 | 1987 | 2.5 |
| | | 1988 | 3.4 |
| | | 1989 | 3.7 |
| 1992 | 87 | | |

[1] Diers (1982), and ACNM 5-year membership surveys through 1992 (Walsh & DeJoseph 1993).
[2] Declercq (1992) National Center for Health Statistics.

midwives' contributions to maternal and child services, as well as of the need for these services, and hence, the imperative to educate more nurse-midwives.

## THE GROWTH OF NURSE-MIDWIFERY EDUCATION

Thus far I have described the demise and then the development of midwifery in the United States, and also the background for the formalization of nurse-midwifery as an extension of public health nursing. The development of nurse-midwifery education continued to be influenced by nursing, and by the professionalization of health care services. By the time the first recognized nurse-midwifery education programs were being developed (1930s), professional nursing in the United States had become established (also as a result of the need for nurses for the war efforts). Nurses had taken the initiative in addressing the quality of maternity care, and were concerned about the adequacy of nursing education both for maternity nursing and as a basis of nurse-midwifery education.

Along with the public health education, considered essential for nurse-midwifery practice, a future-oriented nurse in 1946 advocated that programs for 'clinical specialization' be located within the universities so that the nurse-midwife's or advanced maternity nurse's knowledge would be more adequate and so that these clinical specialists would be 'qualified to work with medical specialists' (Corbin 1946). This perspective of midwifery as a specialized area of nursing practice has persisted, along with the belief that the level of preparation desired should be acquired within the context of a university-based, that is, a professional, education (Blauch 1955, McGlothlin 1964, Anderson 1966).

## Dimensions of professional education

There has been ongoing debate about the scope and level of education that is minimally essential for safe clinical practice, and that is congruent with a professional level and type of competence. According to Schon (1983), education for professional practice not only enables the person to provide competent clinical care, but to interact, that is collaborate, with other health professionals in planning, organizing and studying health care programs and issues.

As nurse-midwives sought to establish midwifery services within the broader context of maternal and child health, they adopted or reflected the strategies that have historically accompanied the establishment of a distinct profession: the formalization of a unique body of knowledge (prerequisite learning and a specific curriculum); control over their education and subsequent practice, and contribution to the specific body of knowledge through research (David 1948, McGlothlin 1960, Anderson 1966, Vollmer & Mills 1966).

Education in basic sciences relevant to professional practice is thought to be a prerequisite to professional education, where one builds on this base and learns to apply knowledge in a more specialized context, often in conjunction with other learners in related disciplines. Thus, special knowledge and skills, unique to the discipline, are acquired, and the new professional is prepared to address the issues that are most relevant to their discipline, as well as to collaborate or communicate with persons who have related societal and/or scientific concerns.

In addition to the 'basic sciences' (i.e. behavioral and biological sciences) that typically accompany professional, university-based, education, the integration of clinical practice and the related theory base was, and is, important in the development of the curriculum for nurse-midwives, as for other professions (Mc-Glothlin 1964). This integration of the 'science', the professional 'knowledge' and its 'application' required that the didactic coursework be combined with clinical practice opportunities. This integration is typically accomplished within the university and its association with practice environments.

As described above, the initial nurse-midwifery education programs were developed along with the establishment of nurse-midwifery services. The students were assured the type and quantity of clinical practice, with qualified faculty nurse-midwives, in both in-hospital and out-of-hospital settings. An early and continuing issue in nurse-midwifery education is how to achieve a balance between the types of clinical settings where students learn.

The initial 'clinical site' for nurse-midwifery practice and education was the expectant family's home or an out-of-hospital birth center, and the nurse-midwife learned to do home births. As nurse-midwifery moved into the hospital environment along with the majority of births, the later education programs were developed in universities and their associated hospital and outpatient clinics. In the public hospital setting nurse-midwives became oriented to hospital and 'tertiary-level' (i.e. high risk) care, but brought a family-centered care perspective to that context.

The contemporary education of nurse-midwives has taken more of a community orientation. Students generally learn in a variety of practice settings, i.e. public and private settings, in-hospital and, if possible, out-of-hospital. Societal and local community needs are involved along with individualized personal care for a woman and her immediate family. This broader orientation is most currently reflected in the ACNM's Board of Directors' position statement, identifying 'Certified Nurse-Midwives as Primary Care Providers' (ACNM 1993d). This description conveys an emphasis on the ambulatory health care of women (and newborns) along with health promotion, education and disease prevention. Thus, *education* for nurse-midwifery was, and is, integrally linked with the maternity as well as women's health *services* that are needed, as is characteristic of a profession.

## Professional organization

The societal service associated with professional practice of nurse-midwives, coupled with a level of technical and theoretical competence, became formalized as nurse-midwives developed a separate professional organization, the American College of Nurse-Midwives (ACNM). The history of the development of the ACNM is summarized in several historical reviews (Shoemaker 1947, Hiestad 1978, Tom 1982, Varney 1987).

In brief, it became imperative for nurse-midwives to form their own professional organization. Neither of the two nursing organizations, the National League for Nursing (NLN) or the American Nurses' Association (ANA), considered midwifery to be nursing (Reinders, cited in Tom 1982). The nurse-midwives did not want to give up their identity with their international midwifery counterparts. Despite their identification with nursing and their deliberate efforts to 'find a place' in either organization, they were unable to retain their identity as both nurses and midwives within either organization. Nevertheless, they thought that it was essential to organize themselves in order to address the critical issues of licensure for practice and recognition of education programs, after the initial efforts to establish nurse-midwifery education and services were successful. Therefore, in the late 1940s and early 1950s, a small group of about 20 nurse-midwives began to set the standards for the practice and education of nurse-midwives. The membership of ACNM in 1992 was 3151 (Walsh & DeJoseph 1993), out of approximately 4500 CNMs.

The American Association of Nurse-Midwives was organized in Kentucky in 1929, and merged in 1968 with the American College of Nurse-Midwifery, which had organized in 1955, to become the American College of Nurse-Midwives. The approval of education programs was initiated in 1962 and in 1982 the ACNM Division of Accreditation was recognized by the US Department of Education as an accrediting agency (ACNM 1991). The examination of graduates of accredited nurse-midwifery education programs was initiated in 1971 (Foster 1986), and mechanisms have been established to discipline certified nurse-midwives as well as to assure their continued competency (Varney 1987). Thus, the dimensions of professional accountability and regulation of its members characterize nurse-midwifery (Schon 1983).

## 'Professionalism' and midwifery

This review documents that American nurse-midwives, at a time when they were accepted by neither medicine nor nursing,

became educated and organized to form an independent association of individuals, dedicated to contributing to the improvement
and provision of maternal/infant health care. These accomplish-
ments should serve as evidence to even non-nurse midwives that
a professional midwifery counterpart has emerged on the other
side of the Atlantic.

It is this 'professionalization' of American midwifery reflected
in the nurse-midwives that distinguishes them from the 'lay
midwives' who have also continued to be a part of American
midwifery (Litoff 1978, Teasley 1986). Some critics of nurse-
midwifery (i.e. of the Certified Nurse-Midwife) (Arms 1975,
Rothman 1981, Teasley 1986) charge that along with 'professionalization', the CNM has lost her/his autonomy by becoming part
of 'the obstetric team' and subject to the influence, if not the
control, of the physician within the hospital domain. In contrast,
lay midwives have sought to establish 'an occupational niche'
outside the perimeter of the physician and the hospital. Teasley
(1986) explains that lay midwives:

Having grown out of the home-birth movement, independent
midwives seek to attend deinstitutionalized births for a self-selected
clientele that advocates the option of *deprofessionalized* [my italics]
maternity care.

She contrasts the 'independent midwives', as those who deliberately 'espoused an ideology of deprofessionalization', with the
nurse-midwives whose

strategy was professionalization and the creation and maintenance of
working relationships with physicians to whom they were legally and
structurally subordinate

In some areas of the United States a coexistence prevails;

implicitly honor(ing) one another's claims to occupational turf,
recognizing that the medical profession, the legislature, and the laity
were (are) the likely arbiters of their respective fates.

(Teasley 1986)

This is an accurate characterization of the current status of the
relationship between CNMs and 'independent' or 'lay' midwives.
The recent meetings (1989 to the present) of the Interorganization
Work Group of ACNM and MANA members reflect many
elements of their common commitments and philosophies. However, it is the issue of 'professionalism', which has different
meanings for the two groups, that at present inhibits real

unification (ACNM 1993e). This is especially evident in the area of professional education, in that ACNM members want to maintain the standards for education which they have established and which are reflected in the Division of Accreditation criteria (ACNM 1991); and the MANA midwives want to maintain their apprenticeship and proprietary or independent school patterns of education (Davis 1981, COMBS 1991). Although prior to and during the earlier part of the 20th century, preparation for the practice of a profession was generally through apprenticeship, or preceptorship (Blauch 1955), these models of education are not considered congruent with contemporary professional education because: 'The knowledge and skill required for practice of a professional are too complex to be transmitted by "apprentice-ship"' (McGlothin 1964, Anderson 1966). There are also differ-ences regarding the appropriate range of practice and the scope of enforcement of ethical standards (which will not be further elaborated). Thus, the issues of 'professionalism' divide 'lay' and 'professional' midwives.

Nevertheless, CNMs have espoused the strategies of profes-sional education in order to educate individuals who have the potential to become full participants in the contemporary system of health care, with the aim of providing quality services to women and infants. The expansion of nurse-midwifery education programs and associated clinical services has continued.

## Education level and types of program

The early organizational activities of members of ACNM included several work groups to address education issues. From an initial 'work conference' on nurse-midwifery education in 1958 to the present, there has been the articulation of a curriculum that was considered to be post-basic nursing and potentially graduate level, ideally leading to a master's degree and associated with an institution of higher education (ACNM 1958, 1967, 1976, 1977, Cranch et al 1973 p 15, Maternity Center Association 1983). The basic nurse-midwifery curriculum is currently reflected in the document *Core Competencies for Basic Nurse-Midwifery Practice* (ACNM 1992).

As indicated above, the initial nurse-midwifery education program, of the Maternity Center Association in 1932, was associated with an institution of higher education (Teachers'

College at Columbia University) because of the scope of the curriculum that was desired. In addition, the prerequisite of public health nursing experience often required that the nurse have a bachelor's degree in nursing. Therefore, it was reasonable to place her continued education within a graduate program where she could acquire a graduate degree. The Frontier Graduate School of Midwifery awarded a certificate to public health nurses who completed the midwifery program. Funding limitations prevented an initial affiliation with the University of Kentucky (Sharp 1983).

The first master's program for nurse-midwives was established in 1947 by the Catholic University School of Nursing Education, in conjunction with the Catholic Maternity Institute School of Nurse-Midwifery, in Santa Fé, New Mexico which had been established in 1945 (Shoemaker 1947, ACNM 1958). The students could complete a 6-month certificate program in nurse-midwifery at the Institute in Santa Fé (which in 1954 was extended to 1 year), or complete Master of Science in Nursing degree, with a major in Maternal and Child Health Nurse-Midwifery, through the Catholic University. These programs closed in 1969 due to funding problems. Nevertheless, they were the prototype of the current certificate-basic programs that also offer the option of a master's degree through their affiliating university.

By 1958 there were six nurse-midwifery programs, three of which offered a certificate and three of which offered a master's degree as well as a certificate (ACNM 1958). All required that the entrant be a nurse, have public health nursing education or experience, and preferably have a bachelor's degree with a major in nursing. By 1965 there were nine education programs (ACNM 1967), and by 1980 the number had more than doubled to 21 with three additional programs in the process of development. Of the 21 programs 13, or 62%, offered a master's degree. The rapid expansion of education programs since 1960 is evident in Figure 7.1, along with the pattern for programs to be graduate level or include a MS option (5 of 10 certificate programs offer this option).

From 1982 to 1988 one education program offered a doctoral degree in nursing science (DNS) as a post-baccalaureate program. Because a doctoral program places an emphasis on research preparation, this course never gained popularity, since nurses seeking nurse-midwifery education are primarily interested in acquiring advanced practice skills with a lesser emphasis on research. As indicated initially, there are currently 40 accredited

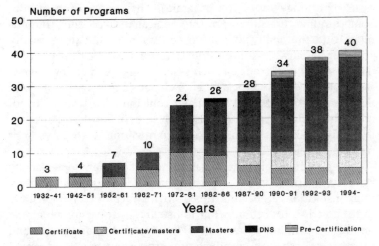

**Figure 7.1**  Net increase of basic nurse-midwifery education programs by decade. (Adapted from Sharp E S 1983 Nurse-midwifery education: its successes, failures and future. Journal of Nurse-Midwifery 28(2): 17–23.)

programs, 28 are master's programs, with 32 of 40 offering a master's degree, or the option of one, for nurse-midwives. In addition, six of the most recently accredited programs are master's-basic programs.

The increase in the number of education programs in the 2 years from 1990 to 1992 is noteworthy; in this period ten new programs were accredited by the ACNM Division of Accreditation. This is as many programs as existed in 1971, 40 years after the first nurse-midwifery education program opened at MCA in New York in 1932. In the 60-year history of nurse-midwifery education, two-thirds of the programs that exist were initiated in the last one-third, or 20 years, of that time. The factors associated with this growth of programs are also those associated with their difficulties and closures.

Of the 50 nurse-midwifery education programs that opened between 1932 and 1990, 24, or nearly half, have closed. Over half of the programs that have closed (13 of 24) were certificate-basic programs, one-third (8) were refresher/pre-certification programs and five (5) were master's-basic programs. In part, these closures represent the tenuous establishment of nurse-midwifery education as well as a pattern for programs to develop, and have more stability, within larger institutions (although that did not always assure the longevity of the program). The continuation of adequate funding, the support of the medical and academic communities, and the ability to acquire and maintain adequate faculty and clinical sites have been critical factors. Although supportive official statements from medical associations, such as the American College of Obstetricians and Gynecologists (ACOG) (Joint Statement 1971, 1975, 1982) have contributed to the ability of more nurse-midwives to practise fully (i.e. obtain hospital privileges for deliveries), tension and competition with physicians remains (Lubic 1982).

Programs have also proved more durable when some faculty staff have earned tenure, a permanent academic position, within their institutions, reflecting the need for faculty to demonstrate the scholarly productivity that is usually essential for obtaining tenure. The multiple demands of teaching, clinical practice and research or scholarly productivity are exhausting, and are a deterrent to CNMs in seeking faculty positions, or are a cause of faculty loss (Sharp 1983, Murphy 1986). A variety of faculty appointments and associations with clinical practice have been developed to address these concerns (Murphy 1986).

Funding for education programs and for students remains a major concern for the profession (Sharp 1983, ACNM 1993c). Currently, the majority of programs depend on funding from the federal government for advanced nurse and nurse-midwifery training (ACNM 1993b). Thus, support from the federal government (at present from the Division of Nursing and the Maternal and Child Health Bureau of the US Public Health Service), as reflected by the early support from the Children's Bureau (which became the Maternal and Child Health Bureau), has been essential for nurse-midwifery to develop and grow.

## CURRENT STATUS, TRENDS AND ISSUES

### Degree and non-degree options

The pattern of both certificate and master's-level programs has continued to the present. In addition to the 'biological and clinical subjects' the graduate degree programs were initially characterized as adding 'teaching in the social, behavioral, and public health sciences' (ACNM 1958). The first report (ACNM 1958) on nurse-midwifery education described the two types of programs this way:

The certificate programs provide adequate training for the practice of nurse-midwifery, whereas the graduate degree programs are oriented toward education for teaching, administration, and research as well.

A recent paper (Rooks et al 1991), addressing nurse-midwifery education, made the following contrast between certificate and master's degree programs:

Certificate programs give their highest priority to preparation for clinical practice, whereas master's degree programs function within environments that emphasize the importance of research and strive also to transmit teaching and leadership skills. Both types of programs are needed.

The implementation of an evaluation and accreditation process, the formalization of the curriculum ('Core competencies'), and the development of the national certification examination, have all contributed to the recognition of the value of retaining both the certificate-basic and the master's-basic programs because both produce competent nurse-midwives (Rooks 1990, Rooks et al 1991). Not only are all programs accredited using the same criteria, and all include the 'core competencies' in their curricula, but the certification exam results are similar for students from both types of programs. The increased demand for nurse-midwifery services, and hence more nurse-midwives, has also been a strong impetus for the retention as well as the expansion of existing education programs.

In addition, the demand for the education of more nurse-midwives has promoted the development of new programs and experimental 'community-based' education. The Community-Based Nurse-Midwifery Education Program (CNEP) established by the Frontier School of Midwifery and Family Nursing is such a program. It is a

'college without walls' . . . a self-paced program that allows students to remain in their home community [and] . . . follow a modular course of study, closely monitored and evaluated by regional coordinators and faculty.

(Treistman 1992)

It retains the linkage with an institution of higher education (Case Western Reserve University), while enabling students to complete most of their coursework and clinical learning experiences within their own community with nurse-midwifery preceptors (Allen 1989). The CNEP is a certificate-basic program with the option of a MS degrees in nursing. It currently has enrolled over 150 students (Treistman 1992), while other programs enrol 8–30 students per year. The duration of most certificate-basic programs is 1 year, and master's-basic programs are 1½–2 years. Although it may take longer (2–3 years) for the CNEP students, who follow a more individualized program of study, to complete their course, this model has the potential for making nurse-midwifery education more accessible as well as more efficient in the numbers of nurse-midwives educated.

Although experience in public health nursing is no longer required, nursing remains a prerequisite to midwifery education. Some master's level programs admit nurses with non-nursing bachelor's degrees, and some admit non-nurses who have a bachelor's degree (Mourtoupalas & Burst 1992). Those students without prior nursing education complete a nursing curriculum prior to the nurse-midwifery portion of the program, and those with a non-nursing bachelor's degree complete the courses required for a BSN prior to the graduate courses in nurse-midwifery if the program offers a MS degree in nursing.

Currently in the US, two-thirds (67.4%) of certified nurse-midwives have a master's degree or higher (in contrast to about one-third of other nursing specialists). Slightly less than 15% have less than a bachelor's degree, and 3% have doctoral degrees (in contrast to less than 2% of nurses) (Secretary of Health and Human Services 1991, Walsh & DeJoseph 1993). Although the current number of nurse-midwives in the United States, 4500, is relatively small, with approximately 250 graduates a year at present, the increase from a total of 500 in 1960 is ninefold.

Thus, a nursing base as well as an emphasis on graduate level education has continued to characterize nurse-midwifery education. There also continues to be a need to retain non-master's level and non-degree programs, such as: certificate-basic, pre-certification programs for foreign-trained nurse-midwives, and a non-degree option within master's programs for nurses who already have a master's degree. This third type of program is also referred to as post-master's education.

The certificate-basic programs enable nurses who do not have a baccalaureate or academic degree to access the nurse-midwifery curriculum. Currently in the United States the majority (70%) of RNs have an associate degree (AD, 62%) or diploma (8%) (Report to Congress 1991), despite the efforts of the nursing profession to require the baccalaureate degree as the minimum qualification for professional nurses. The certificate-basic programs also enable those nurses who have already acquired a master's degree to obtain education as nurse-midwives without earning a second master's degree.

Some master's-basic programs also enrol students who already have a master's degree in nursing as post-MS 'non-degree' students. These students take the courses required in the nurse-midwifery program without repeating what are usually considered to be the additional graduate courses. (These usually include statistics and/or research, general health policy, and nursing theory). Upon completing the nurse-midwifery courses students are eligible for the ACNM certification exam.

Thus, a range of educational options that are post-basic nursing are currently available.

## Doctoral education

One early leader in the organization of nurse-midwifery education anticipated the need for the nurse-midwife educator, clinical specialist or administrator to acquire post-master's or doctoral education, because of 'the complexity of knowledge related to maternal and infant care and the rapidity of its growth' (Shoemaker 1967). This has indeed become the case since doctoral education is now expected of nurse-midwives who hold tenure-track or 'regular' faculty positions within the universities which offer nurse-midwifery programs.

Also, as the curriculum in nurse-midwifery has expanded over the past 35 years to include newborn care, family planning, women's health care, topics related to health policy and research principles, and, most recently, primary care, it has been necessary for nurse-midwives interested in teaching, research and/or administrative positions to acquire preparation for these roles at the doctoral level. Nurse-midwifery programs could not increase the course content and clinical experience related to expanded areas of practice, and at the same time retain courses in teaching, administration or research that went beyond parent education and a more limited research project or master's thesis. Therefore, the focus of programs has become preparation for clinical midwifery practice. In addition, the graduate programs include more emphasis on research, health policy and leadership roles in conjunction with practice issues. Formal or fuller preparation for conducting research or for leadership roles requires further education.

Not only has doctoral preparation become important for faculty staff who hold positions within university-based programs, but the needs of the profession require that a portion of nurse-midwives acquire the skills of scientific inquiry, health policy formulation, education administration and research (Adams 1988, Paine 1991). Contemporary practice requires the use of 'information' of either a numerical or narrative type. Part of the success of nurse-midwifery has been the documentation of positive practice outcomes. However, more research is needed regarding the validity of specific nurse-midwifery care practices. A variety of research skills are called for, that generally require advanced study (Rhodes 1988).

In addition, the need to consider innovative educational models, such as computer-assisted instruction (CAI), community-based education, or alternative patterns of education, requires persons who are prepared to do educational research (Baxter 1980, Paine 1991). Therefore, in addition to the continuing need to prepare more nurse-midwives and more nurse-midwifery educators, there is the need for nurse-midwives with additional specialized skills.

## Advanced nurse-midwifery practice

A final aspect of nurse-midwifery education, that extends beyond basic education, but may not involve doctoral study, is the acquisition of new skills. Among the professional expectations that have been established by ACNM is the requirement of continued education to remain 'current' or competent in practice. This requirement for 'currency' has been formalized by the ACNM Certification Council, which requires the completion of a designated amount of continuing education over a period of time or re-taking the certification examination. Preparation for 'advanced practice' extends beyond this basic competency.

The Clinical Practice Committee (CPC) of the ACNM has established mechanisms for reviewing the addition of various practice skills or clinical procedures to a nurse-midwife's practice (Avery 1992). Recognizing that clinical practice and technology change, the CPC has developed the guidelines for incorporation of new procedures into nurse-midwifery practice which are also incorporated into the ACNM's standards for the practice of nurse-midwifery (ACNM 1987). Such procedures as circumcision, ultrasound, vaginal breech births, use of the vacuum extractor, colposcopy and repair of third- or fourth-degree lacerations, have been reviewed within the context of a nurse-midwife's practice setting. The documentation of need as well as adequate education accompanies this review.

This has implications for the continued educational opportunities that need to be available to nurse-midwives, so that they can be adequately prepared to assume additional responsibilities or carry out procedures in practice settings where this may be necessary. For example, a course on third-trimester ultrasound has been developed at Johns Hopkins University by nurse-midwives for addressing these needs (Paine 1991). At the present time the CPC is working with the Continuing Education Committee of the ACNM to locate and approve high quality courses for nurse-midwives on some of the procedures individuals wish to incorporate into their practices (Avery 1992). A 'Home study program' has also been developed through the *Journal of Nurse-Midwifery* (ACNM 1993d). Thus, the practice of nurse-midwifery has continued to expand from basic maternity services, to family planning, women's health, and primary care, to more specialized procedures (advanced practices) that have become common or necessary.

## CONCLUSIONS

Nurse-midwifery has achieved the status of a professional discipline in the United States. It has retained its identity as a specialty practice in nursing as well as its identity with midwifery in an international context. The professional organization has preserved a range of educational possibilites, including certificate and graduate programs, within schools of nursing, public health and allied health sciences. Nurses as well as non-nurses can earn a graduate degree in nursing (MS or MSN) or public health (MPH), or they can obtain a certificate in nurse midwifery as an extension of their education as nurses. (A summary of the characteristics of accredited nurse-midwifery education programs, detailing prerequisites, degree awarded or options available, clinical sites and graduation requirements, is published annually in the *Journal of Nurse-Midwifery*. This chapter relied on the program information published in July/August 1993 (Whitfill & Burst 1993).

Ongoing issues for nurse-midwives include their relationships with nurses, physicians and 'lay' midwives as they retain or modify their professional identity. The most critical contemporary issue is the imperative to educate more nurse-midwives in response to the US crisis in maternity care services (ACNM 1993a,b). In order to do this, existing programs will need to be expanded and new ones must be developed. This will exacerbate the current shortage of qualified faculty, as well as increase the demands on clinical practices to incorporate learners in their services.

The success of nurse-midwives in establishing themselves within the health care system, and in now being viewed as part of the 'solution' to our current need for maternity care services, as opposed to being seen as 'the problem', has in part, reflected the clarity of their purpose, to provide safe as well as satisfying care to childbearing women and their families, and their ability to collaborate with other health care providers to achieve this purpose. This commitment and this ability have been conducive to the development of high quality education programs. These qualities will also be important as US certified nurse-midwives continue to address these educational as well as other professional and interprofessional issues.

REFERENCES

Abbot G 1915 The midwife in Chicago. American Journal of Sociology 20(5): 683–699
Adams C J 1988 Doctoral preparation for nurse-midwives. Journal of Nurse-Midwifery 33(3): 141–143
Allen S 1989 Frontier School of Midwifery and Family Nursing celebrates 50th anniversary. Frontier Nursing Service Quarterly Bulletin 64(4): 2–7
American College of Nurse-Midwifery 1958 Education for nurse-midwifery. The report of the work conference on nurse-midwifery. American College of Nurse-Midwifery, Santa Fé, New Mexico
American College of Nurse-Midwives 1967 Education for nurse-midwifery. The report of the 2nd work conference on nurse-midwifery education. Maternity Center Association, New York
American College of Nurse-Midwives 1976 Report of workshop – directors of nurse-midwifery education programs. Lexington, Kentucky, February 22–24
American College of Nurse-Midwives 1977 National workshop on nurse-midwifery education. ACNM, Washington DC, February 7–8
American College of Nurse-Midwives 1987 Guidelines for the incorporation of new procedures into nurse-midwifery practice. ACNM, Washington DC
American College of Nurse-Midwives 1991 Policies and procedures manual for the accreditation of basic certificate, basic graduate, and percertification programs in

nurse-midwifery education. ACNM Division of Accreditation, Washington DC, p 6

American College of Nurse-Midwives 1992 Core competencies for basic nurse-midwifery practice. ACNM, Washington DC

American College of Nurse-Midwives 1993a Background on the ACNM/MANA interorganization workgroup on midwifery education (IWG). Quickening 24(1): 29–31

American College of Nurse-Midwives 1993b ACNM Division of Accreditation, Washington DC, January

American College of Nurse-Midwives 1993c Report of the national commission on nurse-midwifery education. ACNM, Washington DC

American College of Nurse-Midwives 1993d Statement accepted by the board of directors. Quickening 24(1): 6

American College of Nurse-Midwives 1993e Actions of ACNM Board of Directors, p 21 and Background on the ACNM/MANA interorganizational workgroups on midwifery education (IWG). Quickening 21: 29–31, January/February

American Nurses' Association 1968 Statement of nurse-midwifery. Bulletin of the American College of Nurse-Midwives 13: 26–27

American Society of Superintendents of Training Schools for Nurses 1909 Fifteenth Annual Report. ASSTSN, First, Baltimore, p 38

American Society of Superintendents of Training Schools for Nurses 1911 Seventeenth Annual Report. ASSTSN, First, Baltimore, p 173

Anderson G L 1966 Professional education: present status and continuing problems. In: Henry N B (ed) Education for the professions – the sixty-first yearbook of the National Society for the Study of Education. University of Chicago Press, Chicago, p 3–26

Arms S 1975 Immaculate deception. Houghton Mifflin, Boston

Avery M D 1992 Advanced nurse-midwifery practice. Journal of Nurse-Midwifery 37(2): 150–154

Baker J 1913 The function of the midwife. Woman 's Medical Journal 23: 196–197

Baxter L 1980 Thoughts on nurse-midwifery and research. Journal of Nurse-Midwifery 25(3): 1–2

Becker H S 1966 The nature of a profession. In: Henry N B (ed) Education for the professions – the sixty-first yearbook of the national society for the study of education. University of Chicago Press, Chicago, p 27–46

Blauch L E (ed) 1955 Education for the professions. US Department of Health, Education and Welfare, Washington DC, p 1–17

Bogden J D (1986) Aggressive intervention and mortality. In: Eakin P S (ed) 1986 The American way of birth. Temple University Press, Philadelphia, p 60–98

Breckenridge M 1952 Wide neighborhoods. Harper and Row, New York

Cameron J 1967 History and development of midwifery in the United States. In: McRedmond A (ed) 1967 Can maternity nursing meet today's challenge? Ross Laboratories, Columbus, Ohio, p 11–19

Chafe W 1972 The American woman, her changing social, economic and political roles, 1920–1970. Oxford University Press, London, p 27–28

Chaney J A 1980 Birthing in early America. Journal of Nurse-Midwifery 25(2): 5–13

COMBS (Coalition of Ontario Midwifery and Birth Schools) 1991 Apprenticeship: a complete education for midwives: saving the successful tradition in Ontario. COMBS, Ontario

Conway-Welch C 1986 Assuring the quality of nurse-midwifery education: the ACNM Division of Accreditation. In: Rooks J, Hass J E (eds) Nurse-midwifery in America. American College of Nurse-Midwives Foundation, Washington DC, p 10–13

Corbin H 1946 A nurse looks ahead. American Journal of Obstetrics and Gynecology 51(6): 811–818

Corbin H, Hellman L M 1960 The nurse-midwife in American obstetrics. The Bulletin of Maternal and Infant Health 7(2): 13–17

Cranch G, Sharp E, Wheeler L 1973 Workshop report – responding to the demands for nurse-midwives in the United States. Nell Hodgson Woodruff School of Nursing, Atlanta, Georgia

David D K 1948 The objectives of professional education. In: A report of the proceedings of the inter-professions conference on education for professional responsibility. Carnegie Press, Pittsburgh, p 7–13

Davis E 1981 A guide to midwifery: heart and hands. John Muir, Santa Fé, New Mexico, p 6–18

Declercq E R 1992 The transformation of American midwifery: 1975 to 1988. American Journal of Public Health 82(5): 680–684

DeLee J B 1915 Progress toward ideal obstetrics. Transactions of the American Association for the Study and Prevention of Infant Mortality 6: 114–138

DeVitt N 1979 The statistical case for elimination of the midwife: fact versus prejudice, 1890–1935 (Parts I & II). Women & Health 4(1, 2): 81–96, 169–186

Diers D 1982 Future of nurse-midwives in American health care. In: Aiken L (ed) Nursing in the 1980s – Crises, opportunities, challenges. J B Lippincot, Philadelphia, 267–293

Dye N S 1983 Mary Breckinridge, The Frontier Nursing Service and the introduction of nurse-midwifery in the United States. Bulletin of the American Association for the History of Medicine 57(4): 485–507

Dye N S 1986 The medicalization of birth. In: Eakin P S (ed) The American way of birth. Temple University Press, Philadelphia, p 21–46

Eakin P S (ed) 1986 The American way of birth. Temple University Press, Philadelphia, p 7

Eastman N J 1953–1954 Nurse-midwifery at the Johns Hopkins Hospital. Briefs 17 (6): 8–13

Eastman N J 1958 Preface regarding nurse-midwifery practice. In: Education for nurse-midwifery: the report of the work conference on nurse-midwifery. American College of Nurse-Midwifery, Santa Fé, New Mexico

Eastman N J 1962 Appraisal of obstetrics in the United States. In: Corbin H, Brown I S, Hughes H H (eds) Meeting the childbearing needs of families in a changing world. Maternity Center Association, New York, p 55–62

Emmons A B, Huntington J L 1912 The midwife: her future in the United States. American Journal of Obstetrics and Gynecology 65: 395–396

Flexner A 1910 Medical education in the United States and Canada. Bulletin No 4. Carnegie Foundation for the Advancement of Teaching, New York

Foster J C 1986 Ensuring competence of nurse-midwives at entrance into the profession: the national certification examination. In: Rooks J, Hass J E (eds) Nurse-midwifery in America. American College of Nurse Midwives Foundation, Washington DC, p 14–16

Hall C M 1927 Training the obstetrical nurse. American Journal of Nursing 27: 373–374

Hardin E R 1925 The midwife problem. Southern Medical Journal 18: 347

Harmer B, Henderson V 1955 Textbook of the principles and practice of nursing, 5th edn. Macmillan, New York

Hawkins J W 1987 Carolyn Conant Van Blarcom. Annual report of the ANA council on maternal-child nursing. American Nurses Association, Kansas City, June

Hemschemeyer H 1932 A training school for nurse-midwives established. American Journal of Nursing 32: 374

Hemschemeyer H 1939 Midwifery in the United States. American Journal of Nursing 39: 1181-1187

Hemschemeyer H 1957 Maternity care with the framework of the public health service. Bulletin of the American College of Nurse–Midwifery 2(3): 49-56

Hiestad W C 1978 The development of nurse-midwifery education in the United States. In: Fitzpatrick M L (ed) Hisotrical studies in nursing. Teachers' College Press, Columbia University, New York, p 86-103

Hogan A 1975 A tribute to the pioneers. Journal of Nurse-Midwifery 20: 6-11

Joint Statements on Maternity Care 1971, 1975, 1982 The American College of Nurse-Midwives, The American College of Obstetricians and Gyneocologists, The Nurses Association of the American College of Obstetricians and Gynecologists, Washington DC

Keane V 1959 Maternity nursing problems. Hospital Topics 37: 89

Keane V 1965 Editorial: Where are we going? The Bulletin of the American College of Nurse-Midwifery 10(1): 1-3

Kelly M (ed) 1983 The next fifty years of nurse-midwifery education. Maternity Center Association, New York

Kobrin F E 1966 The American midwife controversy: a crisis of professionalization. Bulletin of the History of Medicine 40: 350-363

Levy J 1918 The maternal and infant mortality in midwifery practice in Newark, NJ. American Journal of Obstetrics and Gynecology 77: 42

Litoff J B 1978 American midwives, 1860 to the present. Greenwood Press, Westport, Connecticut, p 32-42

Litoff J B 1982 The midwife throughout history. Journal of Nurse-Midwifery 27(6): 3-11

Lubic R W 1982 Nurse-midwifery education – the second 50 years. Journal of Nurse-Midwifery 27(5): 5-9

Maternity Center Association 1943 Maternity Center Association, 1918-1943. MCA , New York, p 66

McGlothlin W J 1960 Patterns of professional education. G P Putnam, New York, p 169-170

McGlothlin W J 1964 The professional schools. The Center for Applied Research in Education, New York

Mourtoupalas C, Burst H V 1992 ACNM-accredited nurse-midwifery education programs – program information. Journal of Nurse-Midwifery 37(4): 274-286

Murphy P A 1986 Nurse-midwifery education – challenges ahead (editorial) Journal of Nurse-Midwifery 31(1): 1-2

National League of Nursing Education 1937 A curriculum guide for schools of nursing. NLNE, New York, p 442

Nightingale F 1871 Introductory notes on lying-in institutions. Longmans, Green, London. In: Bishop W J, Goldie S (eds) 1962 A Bio-bibliography of Florence Nightingale. Dawsons of Pall Mall, London, p 96

Noyes C D 1912 The training of midwives in relation to the prevention of infant mortality. American Journal of Obstetrics and Gynecology 66: 1051-1059

Paine L L 1991 Midwifery education and research in the future. Journal of Nurse-Midwifery 36(3): 199-203

Parnall C G 1921 Nursing and the health of the future. Public Health Nursing 13: 577

Parsons E 1921 Child hygiene and public health nursing. Public Health Nursing 13: 285

Reid M L, Morris J B 1979 Perinatal care and cost effectiveness: Changes in health expenditure and birth outcome following the establishment of a nurse-midwife program. Medical Care 17(5): 491-500

Rhodes J M R 1988 Integrating philosophy into the doctoral preparation for nurse-midwives. Journal of Nurse-Midwifery 33(6): 283–284

Robb I A, Dock L L, Banfield M (eds) 1901 The transactions of the third international congress of nurses with the reports of the international council of nurses. J B Savage, Ohio, p 485–486

Roberts J E 1991 An overview of nurse-midwifery education and accreditation. Journal of Nurse-Midwifery 36(6): 373–376

Roberts J 1984 Maternity nursing: historical aspects of clinical practice. In: Fondiller S H (ed) Historical basis of clinical nursing practice in the United States. Conference proceedings, American Association for the History of Nursing, Chicago, p 16–34

Rooks J P 1990 Nurse-midwifery: The window is wide open. American Journal of Nursing 90: 30–36

Rooks J P, Carr K C, Sandvold I 1991 The importance of non-master's degree options in nurse-midwifery education. Journal of Nurse-Midwifery 36(2): 124–130

Rothman B K 1981 Awake and aware, or false consciousness: the cooption of childbirth reform in America. In: Romalis S (ed) Childbirth – Alternatives to Medical Control. University of Texas Press, Austin, Texas, p 150–180

Roush R E 1979 The development of midwifery – male and female, yesterday and today. Journal of Nurse-Midwifery 24(3): 27–37

Schon D A 1983 The crisis of confidence in professional knowledge. The reflective practitioner: how professionals think in action. Basic Books, New York

Secretary of Health and Human Services 1991 Health personnel in the United States – 1991. Eighth report to Congress. Bureau of Health Professions, Health Resources and Services Administration, USDHHS, Public Health Service, Washington DC, p 129

Sharp E S 1983 Nurse-midwifery education: its successes, failures, and future. Journal of Nurse-Midwifery 28(2): 17–23.

Shoemaker M T 1947 History of nurse-midwifery in the United States. A dissertation. The Catholic University of America Press Washington, DC

Shoemaker A A 1967 Curriculum trends in nurse-midwifery. In: McRedmond A (ed) 1967 Can maternity nursing meet today's challenge? Ross Laboratories, Columbus, Ohio, p 57–65

Speert H 1980 Obstetrics and gynecology in America – a history. American College of Obstetricians and Gynecologists, Chicago, p 19

Stern C A 1972 Midwives, male-midwives, and nurse-midwives. Obstetrics and Gynecology 39: 308–311

Stowe HM 1910 The specially trained obstetric nurse – her advantages and field. American Journal of Nursing 10(8): 550–554

Teasley R L 1986 Nurse and lay midwifery in Vermont. In: Eakin PS (ed) 1986 The American way of birth. Temple University Press, Philadelphia, p 246–272

Thomas M W 1965 The practice of nurse-midwifery in the United States. US Department of Health, Education, and Welfare, Children's Bureau, Washington DC

Tom S 1982 The evolution of nurse-midwifery: 1900–1960. Journal of Nurse-Midwifery 27(4): 4–13

Treistman J 1992 Notes from the school. Frontier Nursing Service Quarterly Bulletin 67(4): 3–4

van Blarcom C C 1911 The relation of the midwife problem to the prevention of blindness. Proceedings of the seventeenth annual convention of the American Society of Superintendents of Training Schools for Nurses, May 29–31, J H Furst, Baltimore, p 110–122

van Blarcom C C 1914 Midwives in America. American Journal of Public Health 8(4): 197–207

Varney H 1987 Nurse-midwifery, 2nd edn. Blackwell Scientific Publications, Boston p 19–36

Vollmer H M, Mills D L (eds) 1966 Professionalization. Prentice-Hall, New Jersey

Walsh L V 1991 Midwife – an historical perspective. A brochure to accompany an exhibition on the history of midwifery at the National Library of Medicine, American College of Nurse-Midwives, Washington, D.C.

Walsh L V, DeJoseph J 1993 Findings of the 1991 annual American College of Nurse-Midwives membership survey. Journal of Nurse-Midwifery 38(1) 35–41

Wertz R W, Wertz D C 1977 Lying-in – a history of childbirth in America. The Free Press, New York

Wertz R W, Wertz D C 1990 Notes on the decline of midwives and the rise of medical obstetricians. In: Conrad P, Kern R (eds) The sociology of health and illness, 3rd edn. St Martin's Press, New York, p 148–160

Whitfill K A, Burst H V 1993 ACNM-accredited nurse-midwifery education programs – program information. Journal of Nurse-Midwifery 38(4): 216–227

Willeford M B 1933 The Frontier Nursing Service. Public Health Nursing 25: 9–10

Williams J W 1912 Medical education and the midwife problem in the United States. Journal of the American Medical Association 58(1): 1–7

Ziegler C E 1922 How can we best solve the midwifery problem? American Journal of Public Health 12: 409

# 8

# The re-emergence and professionalization of midwifery in Ontario, Canada

*Holliday Tyson   Anne Nixon*
*Arlene Vandersloot   Kate Hughes*

## THE HISTORY OF MIDWIFERY IN CANADA

Throughout most of the 20th century, Canada has been the only western industrialized country with no legal provisions for the practice and the profession of midwifery. Until the 17th century, European tradition, carried over to North America, established that only women were to be present at birth (Donegan 1979). In the 18th century, it became fashionable among the upper classes to have 'male midwives' or 'male accoucheurs' (Scholtoen 1984), although most areas of North America were too sparsely populated for such trends to take hold until the late 19th century.

## The suppression of midwifery

It was more than a mere fashion trend that resulted in the usurpation of midwives as the primary birth attendants. Midwives were the victim of an interprofessional conflict with a newly created medical profession, formed in North America in the 19th century. Before that time there were many sects of health care professionals; the medical profession dominated largely because of their class connections rather than on account of any technical superiority. They obtained new licensing laws which sealed the medical profession (formerly called 'regulars') as a monopoly and all non-licensed health care workers were essentially outlawed.

## Medical legislation

The first legislation was introduced in Upper Canada in 1795 with the Act to Regulate the Practice of Physic and Surgery (Biggs 1983). It imposed a penalty on any person practising 'physic or surgery' in Ontario without approval from a Board of Surgeons. Anyone practising surgery, physic or midwifery before the passing of the Act was exempt, although this Act did not expressly exempt the 'female midwives', as did some later acts.

The 1795 Act was repealed in 1806 to be followed in 1827 by an Act which imposed a large fine or imprisonment for unauthorized practice. In contrast to the earlier one, the 1827 Act did have an explicit exemption for 'female midwives'. Physicians lobbied the legislature to delete the exemption and in 1839 it became law that any practitioner of midwifery had to be a member of the College of Physicians and Surgeons. This Act, however, was quickly repealed by Queen Victoria herself and the earlier Act, exempting female midwives, remained in force until 1865.

In 1865, the Medical Act was passed which took away the exemption for female midwives and prohibited them or anyone who was not a registered physician, from recovering fees for midwifery. This legislation was not widely supported by the public and there was overt demand from women for birth attendants who were members of their own sex. Despite the takeover by the medical profession of licensing for midwifery, midwives continued to practise both in the United states and Canada. American historians noted that midwives carried on working primarily for black and immigrant populations, and many people believed that opposition to midwives was part of an anti-immigrant and anti-black prejudice (Ehrenreich & English 1973).

## Early support for midwifery

At the time in Canada, publications such as the *Globe* and *Mail* supported midwives. The *Globe* argued that both midwives and physicians made mistakes but the difference was:

The qualified practitioner can generally cover his mistakes with learned explanation and no one has to expose his error. The uneducated woman who loses a patient has all the doctors at once publishing her mistake . . .

(Ehrenreich & English 1973)

## The economic conflict

At the same time physicians were having a difficult time surviving in a new country, where the population was not only sparsely scattered but was not yet dependent on the new medical profession for health care. The economic conflict between doctors and midwives is evident in historical materials (Report of the Task Force on the Implementation of Midwifery in Ontario 1987).

Midwives in Canada continued to practise despite laws prohibiting them from doing so. From 1895 to the present, however, the medical monopoly in Canada has remained substantially unchallenged, despite attempts by the National Council of Women, at the beginning of the 20th century, to have the law changed.

## A tradition of midwifery

During the first half of this century, Canada's indigenous peoples had a strong tradition of midwifery, and there were many midwives living in Canada who had trained formally in the UK, Europe and other countries. Nonetheless, the medical monopoly on childbirth care had developed earlier and was protected fiercely.

After World War II the childbirth issue again arose publicly, and the natural birth movement became popular with a very small minority of the middle classes. Although this movement was essentially antifeminist in its roots (Romalis 1981), it emerged in the 1960s and 1970s as a radical challenge to the established medical profession, and as part of a movement of women who were fighting to gain control over their bodies. Despite lack of professional sanction and public funding, women increasingly continued to demand midwives.

## CONSUMER DEMAND

Throughout the later 20th century, women became increasingly critical of the interventionist approach of medically controlled childbirth. They became concerned about the high rates of caesarean sections; the extensive use of medication; forceps delivery, and the lack of dignity and respect given to women throughout the birth process. The other issues were the disruption of the bonds between the mothers and newborns in the hospital birth, and the lack of attention paid to women's psychological and social needs throughout pregnancy and during the postpartum period.

Episiotomies, elective induction, caesarean sections and the routine use of forceps and drugs became the norm despite the high risks involved in these practices. Many commentators began to feel that obstetrics was on the verge of transforming childbirth into an entirely surgical procedure. A look at the rise in the rate of caesarean sections indicates this was a well-founded fear; in Canada and the United States the caesarean section rate is 14–19% while in countries such as Holland, the rate is 3.8%. Consumers came to see that countries with midwives have superior perinatal mortality statistics (Stewart 1987). Ontario in 1985 had a caesarean section rate of over 25% (Report of the Task Force 1987) and Canada's birth mortality rate ranked fourteenth in the world.

## GROWTH OF MIDWIFERY

It was virtually impossible 15 years ago for a pregnant woman to choose a midwife as caregiver. From 1978 growing dissatisfaction, among women and their families, with Ontario's maternity care system fostered a new willingness to take childbirth matters into their own hands. A small number of women, supported by a few radical physicians and by each other, began to learn to be midwives. Over the next decade, a growing number of women became midwives, patching together often impressive apprenticeship education with opportunities to learn, intern and complete preceptorships in other countries.

Midwives in Ontario have diverse educational backgrounds: the majority are apprenticeship-prepared, some have direct entry formal midwifery education from Britain, Holland or Germany and some have nursing backgrounds. What has been shared from the beginning of working together has been a philosophy of care.

The last 15 years have seen the growth of a midwifery

community, coinciding with some remarkable political processes and events. The Ontario midwives have been supported by the international community of midwives, in particular through the International Confederation of Midwives. This has given them the opportunity to learn from both the travails of different midwifery systems around the world, and from the shortcomings of the Canadian approach to care in childbirth. This has led to a strong vision of an autonomous midwifery profession, clearly separate in education and administration from the profession of nursing; clearly founded on informed choice, continuity of care-giver and choice of the full range of birth settings, and utilizing teachers who are also current practitioners.

# THE PROFESSIONAL RE-EMERGENCE OF MIDWIFERY

## The Ontario Midwifery Task Force

The Task Force on the Implementation of Midwifery in Ontario, set up in 1986, published an extensive report in 1987 recommending the licensing of midwifery as an autonomous profession with its own College of Midwives. The Task Force members travelled throughout Ontario listening to individuals and organizations about the birthing process; there were more than 500 written submissions, and oral presentations on behalf of 180 organizations and individuals. Midwifery care facilities in the USA, UK, Denmark and Holland were visited (Task Force 1987)

Midwives had practised openly in Ontario since the late 1970s despite the lack of legal status and despite the fact that their care was not covered by the Ontario Health Insurance Plan. Midwives endured, on a daily basis, the risk of criminal and civil actions, inquests and public persecution by the medical profession during the years they served as practitioners outside the law, providing an alternative to the medical model where birth is viewed as an illness requiring intervention. Despite, and in part because of these hardships, a dedicated profession emerged, with at least half of the practising midwives active in the political work of establishing systems of education and self-regulation.

## The Association of Midwives

In 1994, there are about 150 people active in the Association of Midwives (AOM) with 65 practising midwives in the province. The AOM was founded in 1984 as an amalgamation of lay midwives and nurse-midwives, with a shared vision and willingness to take on a task demanding years of unpaid hard work: the integration of midwifery.

## Legislation for midwifery

Now that Ontario has legislation which gives midwives legal status, a College of Midwives which regulates the profession and a formal education structure through Ontario universities, the situation for midwives will be dramatically altered. Midwifery in Ontario to date has been an almost exclusively women's profession, with a feminist philosophy including the principle of choice. In almost all of Canada, to practise as a midwife has meant to risk legal action such as the charge of practising medicine without a licence, and criminal negligence.

In 1994, midwifery is on the threshold of being integrated into the Canadian health care system. Legislation for midwifery was introduced in 1991 and came into effect at the end of 1993; universities began to provide the first Canadian programmes, and an interim governing body (currently the Transitional Council of the College of Midwives) has been functioning for several years.

## THE ONTARIO PHILOSOPHY OF MIDWIFERY

Midwifery in Ontario has been founded by a strong coalition of childbearing women and midwives, who together develop the principles of informed choice and respect for birth as a normal life event. The woman herself is the central and important person during childbirth. Every woman has the right to make informed decisions about where, how and with whom she will give birth. This credo is fundamental to what midwives in Ontario value in midwifery.

The following statement of philosophy has been adopted by the Transitional Council of the College of Midwives concerning midwifery care:

• Midwifery care is based on a respect for pregnancy as a state of health and childbirth as a normal physiologic process. Midwifery care respects the diversity of women's needs and the variety of personal and cultural meanings which women, families and communities bring to the pregnancy, birth and early parenting experience.

- The maintenance and promotion of health throughout the childbearing cycle are central to midwifery care. Midwives focus on preventative care and the appropriate use of technology.
- Care is continuous, personalized and nonauthoritarian. It responds to a woman's social, emotional and cultural as well as physical needs.
- Midwives respect the woman's right to choice of caregiver and place of birth in accordance with the Standards of Practice of the College of Midwives. Midwives are willing to attend birth in a variety of settings, including birth at home.
- Midwives encourage the woman to actively participate in her care throughout pregnancy, birth and the postpartum period, and to make choices about the manner in which her care is provided.
- Midwifery care includes education and counselling, enabling a woman to make informed choices.
- Midwives promote decision making as a shared responsibility, between the woman, her family (as defined by the woman) and her caregivers. The mother is recognized as the primary decision maker.
- Fundamental to midwifery care is the understanding that a woman's caregivers respect and support her so that she may give birth safely, with power and dignity.

## THE ESTABLISHMENT OF MIDWIFERY

So, how is the establishment of this woman-centred midwifery profession being achieved? More importantly, what are the challenges and risks which come with integration into the health care system? The story of midwifery in Ontario is a story of women seeking choices, who became an organized and articulate coalition for change. It is also about midwives who learned from observing the progress and institutionalization of midwifery in other countries where midwifery is the status quo; a commitment to midwifery must be accompanied by a commitment to and competence in political work, in the realm of legislative, educational and health care institutions.

Midwifery has re-emerged in response to public demand in many parts of Canada and the United States, but it is only where there have been political opportunities for the profession to re-establish itself legally, that midwifery practice has increased, and a midwifery community has developed. It is important to challenge the idealization of lay midwifery which can impede the process of recognizing and compensating midwives, and making their care accessible to women, by a romanticized view of the unregulated, independent, privately funded midwife.

In Canada, midwifery has flourished and been publicly supported only where there is the potential for legal recognition and public funding. Unlegislated midwives have been subject, not to lack of regulation, but to a form of punitive overregulation. This has been in the form of persecution through court cases, inquests and public harassment by medicine and nursing. Women wishing to become midwives have had to be superwomen, making rare personal connections with practising midwives in order to have access to apprenticeships. They have had to cope with systematic medical opposition, to be willing to manage without an income and to be unpaid attendants at births for 2–5 years, being available at all times to the midwife-teacher.

## Development of legislation

It was the opening of the Health Profession Legislation Act in 1983 (a process which only occurs about every 15 years) that provided an opportunity for midwives to convey their case and their vision for legislated midwifery to provincial government. Fortunately, midwifery consumers had developed a group with more than 1000 members to support midwifery legislation: the Midwifery Task Force of Ontario. Midwives had formed a professional association and were in the process of amalgamating the Ontario Association of Midwives (practising midwives from a wide variety of backgrounds) with the Ontario Nurse-Midwives Association (nurse-midwives who were not practising) into the Association of Ontario Midwives, with a unified vision and concrete goals.

After developing a number of written briefs, meeting with government representatives, and having an independent member's bill introduced to the legislature in 1984, midwives heard the government announce in 1985 the formation of the Task Force on the Implementation of Midwifery, a multidisciplinary group which had a mandate to describe how, rather than consider if, midwifery should be integrated into the Province's health care system.

Their recommendations, following a year of public and professional consultation were published in 1986. These included recommendations for public funding, for multiple routes of entry into midwifery education and for support for the 'follow the woman', small group, continuity of care model which was practised by community midwives in Ontario.

## MIDWIFERY EDUCATION

By 1989, a Curriculum Design Committee was being funded by the Ministry of Health to identify the core components of midwifery education. For the first time community midwives were formally part of a committee deciding the future of midwifery. Together with physicians, nurses, educators, consumers and the invited written input of more than 100 groups and individuals, they made recommendations about the constitution of a midwifery education programme, the admission process, approaches to learning and the selection of appropriate institutions. These recommendations, the *Report of the Curriculum Design Committee on the Development of Midwifery Education in Ontario* are available free of charge from the Ontario Ministry of Health.

They were:

- that a 4-year baccalaureate programme be developed which can be completed in 3 calendar years,
- that at least 50% of the programme content be clinical practice experience, and
- that the practice experience be gained in the context of continuity of care,
- that the admission process prioritize mature candidates with a demonstrated commitment to serving their home community,
- that distance learning be utlized to minimize time away from home for midwifery study,
- that the midwifery faculty be required to be in current practice in the full range of birth settings.

The greatest debate centred on the choice of a university degree for midwifery education. Midwives and consumers shared a concern that this setting could easily lead to overprofessionalization and to an academically oriented midwife, rather than to the 'hands on' midwife who learns in an apprenticeship model and values community practice.

It was agreed, however, that in order to practise autonomously, with hospital admitting and discharge privileges in the Ontario health care environment, midwives would need a university degree. In addition, there was a desire to open research to midwives in a way that would not be possible without a university affiliation.

## The pre-registration programme

One of the recommendations of the Curriculum Design Committee was that a mandatory pre-registration programme be developed, to provide a review of academic midwifery content and an assessment of both theoretical and clinical skills for the currently practising midwives. It was recognized that many of these midwives may become the first midwifery faculty and clinical teachers in Ontario. Midwives supported the concept of a short review and assessment programme as being in the public interest, as well as being helpful to midwives in preparing to become publicly funded primary health care providers.

This programme, funded by the Ministry of Health operated on a one-time basis, with midwife examiners from Holland Denmark, the UK and New Zealand. Of the 74 midwives who entered this programme, 62 successfully completed it and were able to apply for registration with the Transitional College of Midwives.

It is important to acknowledge that in the midst of the success of the midwifery movement, the transition to a new working environment, professional status, government funding and regulation was for many midwives a very painful and unsettling process. What outside observers might assume was a time of pride and satisfaction was for many midwives a period of insecurity and deep reflection on their abilities and their vision.

Midwives with qualifications from other countries who wish to work in Ontario will be able in the future to approach the College of Midwives to determine what orientation to Ontario midwifery and assessments are required to become registered as a midwife.

## THE COLLEGE OF MIDWIVES

In 1989, the Interim Regulatory Council of Midwifery (the precursor of the College of Midwives) was formed. Although the College of Midwives will in time be composed of a majority of consumers and midwives, it was seen as not being in the public interest to have midwives, on the Interim Council prior to legislation.

A liaison committee with many midwives from the Association of Ontario Midwives was formed, and in this way midwives were able to participate in the process of developing standards, regulations, core competencies and a code of ethics. It was invaluable for this process that the Association of Ontario Midwives had already developed prototypes of many of these documents, and the Association's input was respected.

## NATIVE MIDWIVES

Native midwives in Ontario have been granted exemption from the Midwifery Act, in keeping with the spirit of and support for the development of self-government for First Nation peoples. This means that while native women may choose to become registered as midwives, they may practise midwifery among native people in accordance solely with their own regulations under native self-government.

## INDEMNITY INSURANCE

An important factor in self-determination for Canadian midwives has been their success in negotiating professional liability insurance, prior to legislation, including coverage for home birth attendance. This has placed midwives in an advantageous position when discussing hospital protocols and admitting privileges with physicians and nurses.

In North America, the need for midwives to be knowledgeable about professional liability issues and to plan ahead for insurance cover has been a crucial element of success and professional autonomy.

## IMPLICATIONS OF LEGAL MIDWIFERY

Many midwives in Ontario admit both to elation at the long-awaited legal recognition of our profession and deep concern about the fragility of aspects of the kind of care we value.

Clearly, publicly funded and regulated midwifery means that for the first time midwifery care will be widely accessible to women, and midwifery education will be more accessible to those who wish to become midwives. Each year graduating midwifery classes will provide 30–40 midwives, which is more than the total number of midwives who were prepared solely by apprenticeship in Ontario over the last 15 years.

Nonetheless, hard questions must be addressed. As midwives become part of the health care system, will the ability for objective criticism still survive? Will midwives still be able to examine the health care system, professionalism, and primary accountability to childbearing women rather than to institutions? Is the key to the impact of being part of the health care system to be found in the process and progress of the profession of midwifery? The following questions need to be examined rigorously throughout the coming years:

- Who is chosen to become a midwife?
- Who is chosen to help students learn?
- How do we ensure that teachers and regulators of midwifery practice are also practitioners?
- How do we promote the involvement of consumer groups in teaching and assessing student midwives?
- How do we protect and build on the coalition of consumers and midwives which made legislation possible and crafted the model of practice?
- How do we remain committed to keeping apprenticeship as the strong core of the relationship between midwives and student midwives?
- How do we embrace innovative adult learning models?
- How do we introduce student midwives, first into the home setting and later to the hospital setting?
- How do we keep the commitment of each registered midwife to remain competent and confident attending birth in all settings?

## CONCLUSION

There are many observers who believe that it is impossible to maintain the vision of midwifery that has guided midwives and the women they have served over the last decade of struggle for change.

It is important to recall that few observers or authors believed in the 1980s that midwifery as a profession separate from nursing would be possible to achieve; that legislation would allow for and protect home birth; that professional liability insurance for midwives attending home births would be achievable, or that a university would want a midwifery programme other than as a postgraduate course for nurses. All this has been achieved. For midwives in Ontario, and for childbearing women, the work, 15 years later, has only just begun, but we can and should take pleasure in some victories and the earned conviction that we are moving in the right direction.

REFERENCES

Biggs L 1983 The case of the missing midwives: a history of midwifery in Ontario from 1795–1900. Ontario History 75(1): 21–35

Donegan J 1979 Women and medicine: medicine, morality and misogny in early America. Greenwood Press, Westport, Conn

Ehrenreich B, English D 1973 Witches, midwives and nurses: a history of women healers. Feminist Press, Old Westbury, NY

Scholtoen C 1984 On the importance of obstetric art: changing customs of childbirth in America, 1760–1825. In: Leavitt J W (ed) Women and Health in America. University of Wisconsin Press, Madison, p 145

Report of the Task Force on the Implementation of Midwifery in Ontario 1987 Appendix 1. A history of midwifery in Canada

Romalis 1981 Childbirth alternatives to medical control. University of Texas Press, Austin

Stewart D 1987 The five standards of safe childbearing. NAPSAC Publications, Marble Hill, Missouri

# SECTION 3

# Models of midwifery and models for midwifery

# 9

# Models of midwifery in the United Kingdom

*Chris Midgley*

## INTRODUCTION

In order to consider some of the issues surrounding the uptake of models in midwifery, it is useful to look at some of the background relating to the education and training of midwives in Britain.

Student midwives have traditionally been registered general nurses (RGN) until recently. This has meant that student nurses have been socialised into the role of caring for patients who are ill. These nurses then transfer to student midwife status, and the model for care is transferred with them. Davies & Atkinson (1991) identify this transfer of models:

Nursing has traditionally followed the medical model. By bringing into midwifery the same model it may be that the British midwife is in danger of losing that unique role, and the independent practitioner status so proudly proclaimed throughout the world.

## BACKGROUND

### Traditional training and care

Until recently the education of students was based on the apprenticeship model of learning. This model could also encourage the perpetuation of traditions, rather than the rational, systematic, research-based approach which should be exemplified in the mentorship role. The current practice of clinical mentorship of students does not necessarily eliminate the continuation of traditions.

An example of the didactic method of teaching can be found in an early edition of a textbook for midwives (Myles 1953):

Immediately after labour the woman lies in the recumbent position, usually under the influence of a sedative, until she is rested. There is no reason why she may not lie on either side, except that when on her back the uterus is in the mid-line and the lochia drain better. . . The bladder should be emptied, the vulva swabbed and the baby fed, prior to lying in the prone position.

Reading this text 40 years later, may well bring a smile to midwives' faces. Issues such as the individuality of women and questions regarding sedatives, swabbing, positioning of women, and routines in relation to the baby and the mother, could all be regarded as causes for concern about the approach described above. Midwives in Britain might identify these issues but nevertheless, is individualised care substituted for routine care in all circumstances? If individualised care is claimed, what framework, if any, is in place for that care?

Sadly, in some aspects of care, midwifery continues to be at the traditional level. One example of this comes from small study by Blankson et al (1991) on weighing the placenta:

22% of 110 midwives weighed the placenta because it was hospital policy and a further 12% because there was space in the notes.

## A framework for care

Some midwives have already moved away from the traditional model of care, and others are also going in that direction. When the medical model is rejected, what is there to replace it? In Britain midwives claim to practise individualised care. Hospital and community midwives are adopting the concept of team care where smaller groups of midwives are taking responsibility for women from the commencement to the completion of care. Whether team or any other type of care is given, a philosophical framework for care needs to be developed. Otherwise care is based on the individual views of the midwife and possibly of other care professionals.

Frameworks, or models for care, will provide one means of

individualising midwifery care but these have not been over-whelmingly adopted in British midwifery. In a study undertaken by Midgley (1988) questionnaires about the use of models were sent to 145 schools of midwifery in England, with the following results:

The response rate was 93% (135 responses). There was a total of 19 schools who were using nursing models in the education and training of student midwives. The model most frequently used was Orem Self-care Model, followed closely by Roper, Logan and Tierney Activities of Living Model. The reasons given for not using a model were, it is unsuitable for midwifery practice, and models are based on illness whereas midwifery is concerned with health. Others stated that a suitable model for midwifery had not been written.

Since this time, Henderson (1990) has identified a 'Human needs model for midwifery, based on the work of Maslow (1971)'. In outlining the framework of the model Henderson (1990) writes:

Any model should address four areas, the person receiving care, health, nursing (in this case midwifery), and the context in which care takes place. The mother and baby are central to the model. All care given by the midwife has the prime purpose of meeting the individual needs of mother and baby. These needs can be categorised into four essential groups; physical; psychological, including spiritual; social; and educational. Failure to meet the needs of the mother and baby could cause them to regress in all four spheres.

This model has not been widely accepted by midwives.

## THE ADVANTAGES OF USING A MODEL

Advantages to some groups of people may be disadvantages to others. The advantages of using a model will be considered with regard to women, midwives and the learners, the midwives of the future.

## THE WOMAN

When using a framework of care the woman's views need to be defined first. The midwifery care is then developed around the woman's expectations, choice and lifestyle.

In the Orem self-care model, the woman could specify the care she could undertake for herself and, postnatally, for her baby (Orem 1980). The Roper, Logan & Tierney model would enable the woman receiving midwifery care and the midwife to identify the activities of living for the former individual. The woman could then describe the ways in which she carried out her activities of living, and the midwife would develop the framework of care around these activities. The midwife and woman would identify where care was required, and the midwife would then act as the agent for that care. Both of these models put the woman at the centre of care, and encourage her to define her own choices and lifestyle first.

This pattern of care is not available to all, as the House of Commons Select Committee on Health (1992) reported:

Too often they [women] experience an unwillingness on the part of professionals to treat them as equal partners in making decisions about the birth of their child.

Are women in Britain ready and able to make their choices of care? In recent years birth plans have been introduced to enable women to select certain aspects of care during labour. Birth plans vary in design; some point the woman in the direction of certain types of care where she can make a choice, but the freedom to choose may not be available in every matter concerning labour and delivery care. Other birth plans are designed on a more flexible basis. The midwife needs to spend time with the women and her partner, in order for birth plans to be completed. At times blank birth plans are returned. This may be the woman's choice, or it may indicate a need for assistance in order to complete the plan of care.

In Britain at present the Government is attempting to move away from the philosophy of institutionalised care (the 'nanny state'), to the concept of responsibilities and decisions being taken by the individual. This includes the belief that people should be able to make a wide variety of choices for themselves. Example of this are, the sale of state (council) houses to the tenants, thus making these people responsible for their own homes. Other examples are giving parents information about and encouraging them to make a choice concerning the school they wish their children to attend. With regard to health care, the Patients' Charter published by the Government in 1992 states:

The Charter standard is that all health services should make provision so that proper personal consideration is shown to you, for example by ensuring that your privacy, dignity and religious and cultural beliefs are respected.

In order to show personal consideration for the individual, the midwife needs to know the wishes of that person. This applies not only to the aspects identified in the Patients' Charter, but in all aspects of individual care.

In any situation where choice is to be exercised, a person needs to be in possession of the relevant facts in order to exercise the right to choose. The woman needs to know the range of choices available to her. Take for example, a woman's choice between home or hospital admission for labour and delivery. In Britain, women may not be informed that they have a choice in this matter. Decisions may be made on their behalf. If midwives are not giving the women the appropriate information regarding a choice, are midwives acting as autonomous professional practitioners? If either the Roper, Logan & Tierney model, or the Orem self-care model is used, the responsibility of care is firstly the woman's . Her choices come first, and the midwife would have difficulty in proposing midwifery reasons for hospital-based care in circumstances where this was unnecessary.

## The midwife

### Identifying the woman's choices

The use of a model for care can assist the midwife in identifying the mother's individual choices. When information about these is documented, it facilitates continuity of care between midwives, because the women is the central focus of the care.

Furthermore, well documented information aids the woman, if she has access to the notes, and also helps the learner.

### The questioning approach

The framework of a model encourages the questioning approach which is a prerequisite to research-based midwifery care. Using the Orem self-care model as an example, the midwife would be constantly asking whether the woman could care for herself in this particular circumstance. Such questioning may assist the midwife to reduce the wholesale acceptance of approaches to care used in the past.

### Individualising care

Midwives in Britain may have some difficulties with the concept of individualising care. This may at times be due to the hierarchical system of the National Health Service and the concurrent anxiety about stepping out of line. Midwives may also consider they need to conform to society's image of the midwife which is aligned with the nurse/doctor hierarchy. Until recently school education has tended to encourage conformity. Careers advice regarding nursing would only be given to girls, and only to those at a certain academic level of education, who were not necessarily aspiring university entrants. Education within the National Health Service still favours the conformist type of person, in nursing, midwifery and medicine.

Against this background, it is hard for the midwife and the woman receiving the services to identify individual needs. The midwife will find difficulty in encouraging women to freely articulate their needs if the midwife feels constrained in practising as an autonomous professional. The woman may have difficulties if her education was characterised by a conformist approach towards 'authority'.

The largest professional organisation for midwives in Britain, the Royal College of Midwives, is quoted in the Report of the Select Committee on Health (1992) as stating:

Currently women have little choice as to who provides care and the number of professionals involved can reduce the continuity of care which evidence shows does much to promote a good outcome to pregnancy and childbirth. Duplication of care leads to unnecessary intervention and is wasteful of resources.

Furthermore, in the Code of Professional Conduct for the Nurse, Midwife and Health Visitor (United Kingdom Central Council 1992), a new clause states that these professionals should

Work in an open and cooperative manner with patients, clients and their families, foster their independence and respect their involvement in the planning and delivery of care.

Both these statements are dated 1992, when professional organisations in Britain are still attempting to encourage the concepts of individualised care.

## Total care

Midwives often claim to provide total care of the mother, baby, and family, but this is not always seen in practice. In Britain the midwife can visit the woman up to 28 days after the birth of the baby. More often it is the health visitor who visits after the first 10 days. If the activities of living model was used, the midwife could identify reasons for continuing her care. Relevant activities could include, for example, sleeping, maintaining a safe environment, communicating, mobilising and expressing sexuality.

Identifying midwifery care is not a luxury, it is a necessity when human resources are expensive and managers must look at ways of cost-cutting. If midwives cannot identify the care they are giving, then someone else may be chosen to give that care.

## The student midwife

The education which student midwives receive is highly dependent on the role model provided by the clinical midwife mentors. When students identify a conflict between the educational and the clinical philosophies, this is a cause for discord. The educational beliefs may be those contained in current literature, but not those implemented by the institution. Students need to learn midwifery skills. Often they criticise midwifery care as being confusing because of the differing views of individual practitioners. This criticism is particularly relevant when those views are not research-based. As midwifery training takes place in a context of higher education, students are spending less time in the clinical areas. They need an approach to care, therefore, which is readily identified, and ideally an approach which can be transferred to a variety of situations. Frameworks for care offer this.

The education of students has developed to include specific subject areas such as sociology and psychology. These subjects need to be united with midwifery practice. Models identify sociological and psychological issues within their framework.

In order for a model to be used, a comprehensive history needs to be taken to identify the woman's activities of living and her abilities to care for herself. This history-taking involves time as well as communication skills. It is valuable in identifying the woman's views, thoughts, anxieties and choices. At times, these may be unheard. Some British midwives have developed their own midwifery records of care. Where these are used, the student midwife has a resource for identifying midwifery care. Midwifery records also act as a useful tool for research into midwifery care.

## THE PLANNING OF CARE

Where a framework for care is used, the nursing (midwifery) process is the means by which the care is planned. Some British midwives have found difficulties with the process because of their background of nursing. Assessment of needs tends to be regarded as the identification of medical problems, rather than seeing needs from the woman's perspective.

The evaluation of care causes further difficulties. This may be due to the apprenticeship approach to education. The implementation of care at times reflects the apprenticeship model, with all women being given very similar patterns of care. The care given may be related to the number of days since the woman delivered the baby, again reflecting the medical model.

In Britain frameworks for care are rejected because they are seen as too rigid and prescriptive.

## ANALYSIS OF A MODEL OF CARE

The model chosen for analysis is the Roper, Logan & Tierney Activities of Living model. This was proposed by a group of nurses in Edinburgh, Scotland.

The activities of living are identified by Roper et al (1985) as: 'maintaining a safe environment, communicating, breathing, eating and drinking, eliminating, personal cleansing and dressing, controlling body temperature, mobilising, working and playing, expressing sexuality, sleeping and dying'. The latter activities can be applied to midwifery care from preconception to the end of the postnatal period.

If the activities of living were applied to antenatal history taking, the midwife would obtain more information than by using the medical model. Collecting more information however is not necessarily advantageous. The quality of the information is far more relevant than the quantity.

Looking at the 'safe environment' concept of the activities of living, and relating this to pre- and antenatal care, antenatal screening could be justified on the basis of a safe environment for the fetus. This argument may not be completely tenable. The mother may be more anxious following screening; false-positive results may occur causing further screening and anxiety. If screening is not classified under the 'safe environment' heading, what is it identified as, and does it matter?

The preceding points may appear somewhat academic but if midwives choose this framework for care, then these issues will need to be addressed.

Antenatal screening of the blood pressure, urinalysis and abdominal examination is carried out by the midwife. These could again be justified on the basis of maintaining a safe environment. What the midwife needs to identify is how often these observations should be carried out and where. After all, the model is encouraging the continuation of the woman's individual activities of living. The midwife needs to fit in around the woman's other activities.

In labour the activities of living such as communicating, eating and drinking, eliminating, mobilising, and personal cleansing and dressing are all relevant. The woman's own home is the place where these activities are likely to be carried out to her individual requirements. The model therefore reflects the potential for most women delivering their babies at home. The maternity services at present are not organised around home-based care, and do not have the required resources for large numbers of home births.

In some cultures the woman is encouraged to stay in bed for a few days following the birth of the baby. Other women in the family then take over her responsibilities. If midwifery care is encouraging individuality, does the midwife encourage staying in bed, or early ambulation? The model would not be expected to answer these issues, but such questions need to be raised, if an individualised approach to care is selected.

## INDEPENDENT MIDWIVES

In Britain there are a few midwives who work independently of the National Health Service (see Ch. 2). These midwives have an individualised care approach to women and their families. The independent midwife uses the framework for midwifery care that many other midwives aspire towards. As British midwives have rejected the identified frameworks for care, perhaps the independent midwife model could be analysed, described and implemented. Independent midwives appear to spend more time with each woman than do National Health Service midwives. Time means cost and the appropriate number of midwifery personnel would need to be employed.

## CONCLUSION

British midwives have a long tradition of practice. Their history and status has had an influence in other parts of the world. At present there are many changes taking place in midwifery education, and in the National Health Service. There is much that is encouraging, for example the development of midwifery research, and in the recommendations of the House of Commons Select Committee Report, published in 1992. In order to achieve these objectives, midwives in Britain need the education and enthusiasic input which can be engendered by meeting with their colleagues from all parts of the world. The care of women and families is an exciting and important responsibility for midwives worldwide.

REFERENCES

Blankson H, Close B, Couzens P, Maskell K, Thomas M 1991 Weighing the placenta – a questionable practice? Modern Midwife 1(2): 19–21
Davies R M, Atkinson P 1991 Students of midwifery: 'Doing the Obs' and other coping strategies. Midwifery. Churchill Livingstone, Edinburgh, vol 7, p 113–121
Department of Health 1992 The Patient's Charter Rights. HMSO, London, p 12
Henderson C, 1990 Models and midwifery. In: Salvage J and Kershaw B (eds) Models for nursing. Scutari Press, London, vol 2, p 60–61
Maslow A 1971 Motivation and personality, 2nd edn. Harper and Row, New York
Midgley C 1988 The use of models for nursing in midwifery training hospitals in England. Unpublished study, Huddersfield Polytechnic, Huddersfield
Myles M F 1953 Textbook for midwives. E & S Livingstone, Edinburgh, p 451
Orem D E 1980 Concepts of practice, 2nd edn. McGraw-Hill, New York
Roper N, Logan W W, Tierney A J 1985 The elements of nursing, 2nd edn. Churchill Livingstone, Edinburgh, p 20
Select Committee on Health 1992 Second Report. Maternity Services. (Chair Winterton N.) HMSO, London
United Kingdom Central Council for Nursing, Midwifery, and Health Visiting 1992 Code of Professional Conduct, 3rd edn. UKCC, London

# 10

# Hospital-based midwifery projects in Canada

*Sheila Harvey    Karyn Kaufman    Alison Rice*

## INTRODUCTION

Midwifery in Canada is undergoing a dramatic evolution. Only 20 years ago there was almost total suppression of midwives, whereas now legislative reform to make midwifery legal and part of the government-funded health care system is in progress in several provinces. The revival of interest in midwifery represents a challenge to the conventional, medically dominated system of childbirth care in Canada. Although there is a universal quality to the struggles of Canadian midwives and childbirth activists, progress towards the goal of recognising midwives differs from province to province.

The legal situation and features of the Canadian health care system present unique problems and challenges to the inclusion of midwives. Uncertainties about midwives' scope of practice, the ideal organisational practice model, payment method and educational qualifications abound. One model which has emerged is that of midwifery projects located within obstetrical tertiary care centres. In North America, an obstetrical tertiary care centre is a university-affiliated hospital for high risk women and neonates.

## Midwives in tertiary care centres

At present in Canada, there are three examples of a model of midwifery practice within tertiary care centres. These are widely separated geographically and are located in three different provinces: British Columbia, Alberta and Ontario. They share many operational and philosophical similarities and face similar problems, even though they were established independently. Their long-term existence is uncertain because of economic and political conditions and because of the rapidly changing circumstances of the midwifery movement.

Each of the three services is located within a hospital that includes university faculty staff and students from several health professions, most notably nursing and medicine. Although each hospital is a referral centre for women with a variety of medical and obstetrical high risk conditions, and for neonates requiring intensive care, women with normal pregnancies also receive care in these hospitals.

Because midwives were not legally recognised and regulated in any of the three provinces when the midwifery projects were established, each used a mechanism within existing health legislation that permitted specially designated nurses to perform certain functions considered to be medical, such as the delivery of a baby. While this mechanism proved useful in structuring a new model of care and creating awareness of midwifery practice, it has neither resulted in a fully autonomous model of practice nor resolved broader issues of scope of practice and accountability for care.

The remainder of this chapter will describe how and why this practice model came to be established in the three centres. The contribution of the model to the overall development of midwifery in Canada will also be discussed.

## CANADIAN HEALTH CARE FROM 1867 TO THE PRESENT DAY

The British North America Act of 1867 gave provincial governments responsibility for health and education. Each province has responsibility for the health and welfare of its population and, furthermore, regulates health care professionals and provides for their education. The federal government transfers funds to support a system of universal health care coverage known as

Medicare. Because the federal government shares the cost of Medicare with provincial governments, it is able to enforce certain standards and principles which are embodied in federal health care legislation. Provinces must adhere to five essential principles, universality, accessibility, comprehensiveness, portability and public administration, in order to receive federal funding for health care (Torrance 1987).

The introduction of universal hospital coverage in 1948 brought about a proliferation of hospitals and an end to the financial disincentive for a hospital birth. The Medical Care Act of 1966 provided coverage for needed medical care services. These legislative provisions had dramatic effects. They brought health care services into the public domain and ensured access to care for all Canadians. An unfortunate effect, however, was the exclusive focus on hospitals as the place of care and on physicians as the primary care providers. Most other heath care providers, including nurses working in obstetrics, became hospital employees.

Although midwives were part of an informal network of care providers in many areas of Canada until late in the 19th century, they were in no position to organise and resist the transformation to institutional and medical structures (Barrington 1985). As informal networks were replaced by formal, legislated systems, midwives virtually disappeared. By the middle of the 20th century, the only midwives allowed to function in a legally recognised capacity were those in remote and isolated communities which lacked any resident physician. Hospitals recruited nurses with midwifery qualifications to staff the labour wards. They functioned, however, not as midwives but as obstetrical nurses. Only a few remnants of midwifery practice, most notably in Newfoundland, persisted. Even among the indigenous peoples of Canada, where traditional midwifery had always existed, midwives virtually disappeared. This loss was accelerated by policies whereby aboriginal women have increasingly been transported from their communities to give birth in hospital settings under physician care.

While physicians continue to manage the care of almost all women giving birth in Canada, policy changes are being introduced to reshape this emphasis. Across the country, reports and recommendations from health policy planners and government strategists underscore the desirability of increasing community-based care and decreasing the reliance on hospitals and physicians.

The growing momentum for change is reflected in the inclusion of midwifery on many health reform agendas. Additionally, in some centres there are plans for establishing birth centres and active discussion about arrangements and standards for home births.

## RESURGENCE OF MIDWIFERY

The social changes in the later 1960s and 1970s altered women's views of pregnancy and childbirth. In particular, the women's health movement and childbirth consumerism gave rise to a critique of medicalised childbirth. Many women rejected mechanistic images of women's bodies and expressed the desire to regain control over their bodies (Martin 1987).

Some women sought midwives as the caregivers who would enable them to be genuine participants in their childbirth experiences. Since few midwives were able to practise within hospital settings this almost always meant arranging a midwife-attended home birth. Thus as midwifery re-emerged in Canada it quickly became synonymous with home birth and therefore contentious within the medical community. Midwives who attended home births practised without legal recognition. At first they did so more or less covertly, but as time passed and consumer support grew, their activities became more open.

Increasingly, the efforts of consumer groups, practising midwives, and other health care providers have been directed toward attaining legal recognition and regulation for midwifery. The difficulties in achieving that goal have been numerous. Perhaps the greatest obstacle has been the use of legal instruments to control midwives. Since the early 1980s, coroners' inquests, charges against midwives for practising medicine without a license and, on one occasion, criminal charges have been used by the state for this purpose. Generally, however, 'the value of legalising midwifery and providing specialized training in accordance with international guidelines' (Burtch 1992) has been recognised. Clearly, continued suppression and legal sanctions are not seen to be beneficial to the public or to midwives.

On a more positive note, midwives have organised and conducted concerted lobbying efforts and shaped policy discussion about the future of midwifery. They have constructed regulatory frameworks, written a multitude of reports and documents as well as contributing to public and professional education. At the same time, midwives have continued to make midwifery visible by practising within the limits of their particular situations. Consumer groups have complemented these efforts. They also have lobbied provincial governments and provided a valuable role in public education and in fundraising.

## DEMONSTRATION PROJECTS IN TERTIARY CARE CENTRES

The imperative need for visible midwifery practices also spurred the development of hospital demonstration projects. Each of the present three authors has been part of the implementation team for one of the hospital-based midwifery projects. Within each of the three settings, influential individuals, receptive to the idea of a midwifery project, helped obtain support, approval and sometimes funding. The goals of the demonstration projects were much like those of community midwives: to promote change in the care of childbearing families; to provide care that was responsive to the expressed needs of childbearing women, and to keep midwifery alive. The demonstration projects enabled women who chose to have a hospital birth to experience midwifery care.

In each of the three projects, the midwife is the expert practitioner in the care of healthy childbearing women. The care is woman-centred, responsive to individual needs and based on a philosophy of continuity of care throughout the childbearing cycle. The approach is characterised by promotion of the normal processes of pregnancy and childbirth. For example, midwives avoid routine use of technology and unnecessary interventions. The midwives act as advocates for the women and their families, and have pioneered changes in their respective institutions.

## The Grace Hospital Midwifery Program

The first contemporary, hospital-based midwifery service in Canada began in Vancouver, British Columbia in 1981. Since then the program has been reorganised several times. Despite different arrangements and personnel changes the original family-centred midwifery philosophy has persisted. From the beginning, women, who on initial screening were assessed to be low risk, have been cared for, during the antenatal, intrapartum and postpartum periods by a team of midwives with physician back-up.

### The pilot stage: the Low Risk Clinic

In 1981, two midwives with the active involvement and support of one obstetrician piloted a midwifery model of care for 10 women. This initiative was a result of consumer pressure for midwifery care. The immediate success of this pilot project led to the creation of the Low Risk Clinic, in 1982, within the new Grace Hospital, the tertiary care centre for the province of British Columbia. Four midwives with the backup of four obstetricians organised acceptance of and provision of care for low risk women and their families. The program was very small with the enrolment of only four women a month.

Although this program was not funded as a research project, the situation was that of a pilot project. There were many reasons for this, the most important one being that the Medical Practice Act specifically prohibited the practice of midwifery in British Columbia by anyone other than a licensed physician. Special permission from the medical licensing body, the British Columbia College of Physicians and Surgeons, allowed the midwives to practice without fear of prosecution. In granting permission, the College imposed conditions which restricted any expansion of the service and required that the midwives be directly supervised by physicians. Supervision took the form of chart reviews and physician presence at the birth, as well as the physicians being responsible for the admission and discharge examinations. Physicians were considered to have the ultimate responsibility for the management of the clients. The College also required that the midwives all be registered nurses with a recognised midwifery qualification.

During this phase of the development of midwifery care at Grace Hospital the midwives' work was essentially voluntary. Only one was a hospital employee. The others were in positions in affiliated institutions with appointments which enabled them to participate in clinical practice in the hospital. All four were able to integrate the clinic sessions into their work week. The labour care, home visits and on-call was all unpaid. The physicians were reimbursed for their work through Medicare.

As the program evolved, Grace Hospital formalised its status as a non-funded pilot project. Protocols and policies were gradually developed. During this period the program included the possibility of home visits during pregnancy, for early labour care and in the postpartum period. Most families had at least one home visit that focused on the birth plan.

This rather loose organisational arrangement lasted until 1984, and an evaluation was conducted at that time. An external researcher interviewed clients to assess satisfaction. The women and their partners reported high satisfaction, particularly with the amount of time devoted to their visits. They felt their concerns were addressed and the visits enabled them to get to know all the midwives prior to labour (Carty et al 1985). A small study (Buhler et al 1988) compared quality of care as documented in prenatal records. Records of the midwife clients were compared with case-matched patients of general practitioners. When these pre-natal records were used as a basis of comparison, the midwifery care appeared to be superior.

## The Nurse-Midwifery Service

In 1985, the hospital administration, impressed with the success of the Low Risk Clinic and the continuing demand for midwifery care at Grace Hospital, adopted the model and funded a service, called the Nurse-Midwifery Service. Registered nurses who were already employed as obstetrical nurses in the labour/delivery units, were seconded for part of their time to the Nurse-Midwifery Service and became the primary midwives. The service was expanded to enrol up to six families a month. The midwives continued to be employed primarily as labour and delivery nurses. They were released to attend the clinic sessions, and to make daily visits to women during the postnatal hospital stay. One midwife was always on duty in the labour and delivery unit and therefore available to take phone calls and to care for the enrolled clients when admitted in labour. If labour extended beyond the usual 12 hours shift, the care was handed over to the following on-duty midwife, unless delivery was imminent.

During this organisational phase, family practice physicians, rather than obstetricians, undertook to provide the physician supervision which was still required. In British Columbia most obstetrical care is provided by family doctors. Their direct involvement in the midwifery services was an attempt to gain support from this important segment of the medical community. One disadvantage of this arrangement was the interruption of direct referrals from midwife to obstetrician.

The requests for midwifery care continued to exceed the limits of the program. This problem, combined with the midwives being employed primarily as obstetrical nurses in the labour and delivery unit, meant that the midwives often felt pulled between the needs of the midwifery clients and the demands of the labour and delivery unit. In 1990, the midwives called for a moratorium with the intention of restructuring the program to include funding for full-time midwifery positions.

Outcomes for clients from 1985 to 1991 provided convincing evidence of the safety and quality of care provided by the Nurse-Midwifery Service. Hospital administrators were convinced of the merits of midwifery care within the tertiary care hospital. During that period there were 418 births, 204 to primiparas, 214 to multiparas. There were no perinatal or maternal deaths. Only 17 infants (4.1%) were born at less than 37 weeks gestation. Of these, only one was born at under 32 weeks. A total of 37 women (8.8%) were induced and a further 51 (12.2%) received augmentation during labour. Table 10.1 shows the birth outcomes for all women initially enrolled, including those for women referred for obstetrical management during pregnancy or the intrapartum period. Reason for referral included such high risk factors as placenta praevia, breech presentation and twins (Grace Hospital Midwifery Program 1993).

**Table 10.1**  Birth outcomes for women enrolled in the Grace Hospital Midwifery Project 1985–1991

| Type of delivery | n | % |
|---|---|---|
| Spontaneous vertex | 346 | 82.8 |
| Forceps | 28 | 6.7 |
| Vacuum | 5 | 1.2 |
| Caesarean section | 39 | 9.3 |
| Total | 418 | 100.0 |

## The Current Grace Midwifery Program

The current Grace Midwifery Program began, in 1991, to accept 10 clients a month. With administrative support for becoming an official program of the hospital, funds were, for the first time, allocated specifically for the Midwifery Program. One of the midwives assumed the role of Director. Three others were employed either full- or part-time. By having midwives employed solely to care for midwifery clients, aspects of the original program were incorporated. Home visits were again included for early labour assessment and during the early postpartum period. The aim was for 50% of the women to be discharged within 12–24 hours following the birth. The expectation was that early discharge with home follow-up by the midwives would save the hospital money and thus help defray the costs of the program. An additional feature was a series of parent education classes, designed specifically for midwifery clients, with an emphasis on empowering families and building confidence for labour and parenting (Rice et al 1993).

The Grace Midwifery Program continues to function in the environment of a tertiary care centre. The original philosophy, to offer family-centred care which helps women and their families assume responsibility for their own health and health care, persists. The midwives continue to act as advocates for their clients. Despite a 10-year presence in the hospital, the role of advocate continues to be critical, particularly in the area of informed choice so that women truly make their own decisions throughout the childbearing cycle (Rice et al 1993).

## The McMaster University Medical Centre midwifery project

Interest in midwifery care at McMaster University Medical Centre began in the late 1970s. However, attempts at that time to establish a demonstration project were unsuccessful and lacked sufficient support from the medical and nursing community. Eventually, in the early 1980s a collaborative effort, between hospital staff members and university faculty in nursing and obstetrics, resulted in a pilot project in which labour and birth care were provided by selected nurses from the labour ward staff. As in British Columbia, the licensing body for physicians in Ontario, along with hospital committees, gave approval for these nurses to function as midwives and carry out the following actions as delegated medical acts: assisting women at birth, assessing the newborn, cutting and repairing an episiotomy, if needed, and administering oxytocin on their own judgement. Physicians remained ultimately responsible for the care of women and could change a midwifery decision at any point.

In order to assess the acceptance of this model of care, in

1984–1985, women were randomised to receive intrapartum care either from one of the midwives or a physician. There was no observed increase in labour and birth complications in the midwifery group. Furthermore, there was good acceptance of midwives by the eligible women.

. Beginning in 1985, the midwives were permitted to extend their care to include antepartum and limited postpartum care. An extensive research protocol to evaluate the clinical and cost effectiveness of this more complete model was developed and submitted to a national health research agency. While given approval, the research proposal was never funded.

By 1987 the midwifery project was stable and involved up to eight nurses who were approved for the midwifery role.

### Evaluation of the McMaster project

Two small formal retrospective evaluations of the project were conducted in 1987 and 1988. In both, a systematic review of medical records showed a statistically significant reduction in the use of epidural anaesthesia in women cared for by the midwives. The first report (Kaufman & McDonald 1988) showed an epidural rate of 34% for midwifery clients compared with a 49% rate for the women cared for by physicians ($p = 0.016$). The follow-up assessment (McDonald 1989) showed even lower epidural rates for midwifery clients (26%) and an unchanged rate (49%) for the physicians' patients ($p = 0.002$).

Trends were noted also, in the midwifery group, towards reductions in the frequency of amniotomy, episiotomy and operative delivery. The authors were of the view, however, that further reductions in interventions might not be obtained until there were changes in the legal framework of practice, that would end the need for direct physician supervision and increase the continuity of care for women, so there was greater familiarity between a midwife and client.

### Changes to the McMaster project

Between 1986 and 1991 there were many major events in the province that culminated in the passage of legislation that will establish a self-regulating profession of midwifery. Substantial alterations were made to the McMaster project during 1990–1991, so that it would more closely resemble the features of the midwifery practice model incorporated in the new legislation.

In particular the changes facilitated greater continuity of care. Two small teams of four midwives each were formed. Each client meets the four team members during antenatal visits. On-call coverage within each team ensures that women are attended in labour by a known midwife. Daily visits to the postpartum unit enhance continuity of care. Home visits during the antepartum, intrapartum and postpartum periods are made as appropriate. A small number of women who have preferred to give birth at home have been attended by midwives from the project.

*Interprofessional cooperation*

Increasing numbers of women have been cared for each year. A total of 300 women per year are presently accepted for care, but the number of requests is greater than this.

Women may refer themselves or be referred by a physician. Several family physicians refer women directly to the midwives. Others participate in shared antenatal care whereby the midwife and the family physician work out a schedule of visits so that both are involved in the woman's care. Communication is assisted by the women carrying their own records between the two care providers.

The staff obstetricians at McMaster have been supportive from the start. One acts as the primary consultant to the midwives, but all of them provide on-call consultation and direct care if needed. Over the years, increasing confidence in the midwives has been reflected in the development of collaborative relationships between physicians and midwives. The midwives have become a valuable resource for the teaching of medical and nursing students.

*Future prospects*

The midwifery project faces the prospect of imminent change. The new legislation takes effect at the beginning of 1994 and will regulate midwives as autonomous primary care providers under a new statutory body, the College of Midwives of Ontario.

As this chapter is being written, new practice and payment policies are under development that will permit midwives to admit labouring women independently to hospital and discharge well women and their babies. They may attend birth in hospital, at home or in a few newly created birth centers. Most, if not all, midwives will be salaried members of community health agency groups and will not be employed by hospitals.

The majority of the nurses who have participated in the project have undertaken the necessary activities to meet criteria for registration as a midwife under the new legislation. It is hoped that their history of working within the hospital setting will facilitate the acquisition of hospital privileges. In addition, the interprofessional cooperation gained during the long implementation of this project should be helpful to the integration of newly regulated midwives into the existing health care system.

## The Foothills Hospital Nurse-Midwifery Program

The Foothills Hospital in Calgary, Alberta has a long history of introducing forms of care that are responsive to family needs and desires. Routine procedures, such as perineal shaving, had been virtually eliminated and family participation was encouraged as early as 1980.

It was believed that midwifery, with its basic philosophy of birth as a normal, developmental event for which noninterventive, supportive care is appropriate, could be implemented in a hospital setting and safely provide the kind of care women were requesting. A demonstration project for a nurse-midwifery program was suggested. By 1987, there was enough administrative, medical and nursing support to facilitate the development of a pilot project. The three major objectives of the project were: to provide a new option for women; to evaluate midwifery care provided within the health care system, and to increase the job satisfaction of the participating nurse-midwives.

Fortuitously, this work coincided with a provincial government initiative to enhance the working life of nurses. The Foothills Nurse-Midwifery Pilot Project proposal was funded for 2-years under this initiative. Some additional funds were granted directly by the hospital. In October 1990, a coordinator was appointed to begin preparation for the implementation and evaluation of the project.

### Selection and education of nurse-midwife team

The Foothills Hospital Nurse-Midwifery Program has been implemented in three phases. The first phase, of selection and education of a team of six nurse-midwives, began in January, 1991. Registered nurses, with a minimum of 2 years' recent experience in the Foothills Hospital Labour and Delivery Unit, and an interest in participating in the pilot project were invited to apply. A careful selection process was instigated which considered philosophy, commitment, education, experience, professional development, verbal and written communication skills, and clinical knowledge.

Education of the team included a certification course in the transferred medical functions of delivery, episiotomy and episiotomy repair. Following successful completion of this component, the nurse-midwives undertook a second course to expand their role into antepartum and postpartum follow-up care.

### The nurse-midwifery clinic

The second phase began with the opening of a nurse-midwifery clinic in September, 1991. Up to 10 childbearing women who meet low risk criteria are enrolled per month. The women are seen by one or more of the nurse-midwifery team at each visit throughout their pregnancies and at a 6-week postpartum follow-up visit.

At the first and 36-week visits they are also seen by an obstetrician. This same obstetrician is available during any clinic to the nurse-midwives for consultation or referral, if necessary. When obstetrician care becomes necessary the nurse-midwifery team continues to provide supportive care. Whenever possible women are referred back to nurse-midwifery care when the problem requiring referral is resolved.

The nurse-midwives' rotation is designed so that round-the-clock one of the team is working in the Labour and Delivery Unit. When labour commences, the woman contacts the nurse-midwife on duty and remains in contact until admission to hospital. After admission, all care is provided by the nurse-midwife on duty. The on-duty obstetrician is notified of the woman's admission and imminent birth and is available for consultation or referral as needed.

### The third phase

In January, 1993, Phase III of the pilot project was introduced. This phase includes a special class, conducted by two nurse-midwives, to prepare women and their families for active participation at birth and for discharge from hospital as soon as mother and baby are stable.

The hospital stay of 6–10 hours is followed by daily home visits from a nurse-midwife for up to 5 days. If either mother or baby requires medical treatment, the nurse-midwives consult with the appropriate obstetrician or family physician. As a result of these arrangements, good working relationships among physicians and nurse-midwives have developed.

### Evaluation of the Alberta project

Evaluation of the nurse-midwifery project has been under way since its inception. The job satisfaction of all labour/delivery nurses was assessed before the nurse-midwives were selected, and re-evaluated at the end of 1992. Data analysis to compare the job satisfaction of nurses and nurse-midwives and to compare the job satisfaction of nurse-midwives before and after participation in the project is being carried out.

Funding from the Alberta Association of Registered Nurses was obtained for the development of a proposal by a multidisciplinary team of investigators for a randomised controlled trial of nurse-midwifery care. The trial itself is funded by the Alberta Foundation for Nursing Research and has been in progress since February, 1992. It is hoped to enrol 200 women in the trial, with 100 in the experimental or nurse-midwifery group and 100 in the control or usual health care group. Data are being collected about the safety of health care received and the satisfaction of women receiving care.

### Outcomes of the program

As is expected with new midwifery programs (Flint & Poulengeris 1987), fewer women than could have been accommodated received care from nurse-midwives in the first year. This was partly because many women were unaware of the project's existence, despite the distribution of brochures in the community. In addition, the introduction of the randomised controlled trial meant that half the women who requested nurse-midwifery care were randomised to standard care. Thus, effectively, the number of women who might have had nurse-midwifery care was reduced by half.

A total of 60 babies were delivered in the first year. Five women (8.3%) were delivered by caesarean section, 17 (28%) received epidural anaesthesia and nine (15%) received an episiotomy.

The Nurse-Midwifery Pilot Project will be completed in June, 1994. It is anticipated that 150–170 women will have been included in the randomised controlled trial by that time. The data will then be analysed and the findings made available for use in planning future health care for childbearing women.

# ADVANTAGES AND DISADVANTAGES OF THE HOSPITAL MODEL

## Benefits of the projects in tertiary care settings

The review of these three demonstration projects shows clearly the advantages and disadvantages of the model of midwifery practice developed in tertiary care centres. Generally, the projects have contributed to the momentum of the midwifery movement in Canada. They have given midwifery care more visibility, within academic settings that have national influence. Since tertiary care centres are looked to frequently for guidance about new trends, the presence of the midwifery projects provides some incentive for other communities to consider the inclusion of midwifery care.

A direct benefit of the projects has been the provision of a previously unavailable option for childbearing women. Women who have enrolled in these programs have appreciated particularly the nature of the antenatal and postnatal care. The appointments are longer, there are opportunities for in-depth discussions and family members are welcomed at all times. Women's confidence for giving birth has been enhanced by the assurance that a known and trusted midwife would be present. Many women who have experienced midwifery care have become enthusiastic spokespersons about its advantages.

There have also been benefits for the nurses who have made the transition to a midwifery role. They have learned new skills and renewed old ones. Since all of them were employed in birthing units as obstetrical nurses, the transition to the midwife role has given them a new level of responsibility and broadened their practice. Not only have midwifery skills been enhanced, but participation in the projects has fostered leadership skills, political awareness and research skills.

The location of the demonstration projects in tertiary care hospitals has provided medical, nursing and post graduate learners with an opportunity to observe practising midwives. As these students have moved into positions in the health care system, hopefully they have taken with them positive views and up-to-date images of midwifery practice.

Obstetric health care providers also have learned about the ability of a midwifery model to change usual practice. In the birthing units of these hospitals a noninterventionist approach has been visible for others to observe and even emulate. Some long-standing hospital practices have been successfully challenged. The hospitals have cited the midwifery programs as evidence of their progressiveness and responsiveness to consumer demands for choice.

## Disadvantages of the hospital model

Along with these several benefits, there are continuing disadvantages. In all three settings there is considerable constraint upon the midwifery role. The scope of practice of the midwives is limited. They are hospital employees and, as such, are bound by the policies and bylaws of the institutions. Some hospital requirements, such as a fetal monitoring strip on admission to the labour ward or restricting food for labouring women, cannot be avoided easily. Working arrangements are further constrained by contracts that were designed for nurses' working conditions and do not provide the flexibility needed by midwives.

One large obstacle to full implementation of a midwifery role has been the lack of separately funded positions that would free the participating midwives from functioning in two roles: being a nurse and midwife, sometimes simultaneously. Only in the Grace Midwifery Program are the midwives employed exclusively for the program and it took 10 years to establish this arrangement. At McMaster and Foothills this step has not been accomplished. In these two hospitals the midwife on any given day may provide nursing care for a high risk woman in labour as well as be the midwife for her own client in labour. These situations create inevitable tensions within the labour ward.

The major difficulty in all three of the projects is the lack of a legally defined midwifery role that would provide a clear distinction from obstetrical nursing. The reality that the final responsibility for the care of the women and their babies still resides with physicians is the most serious impediment to the full realisation of the role of the midwife. This is not satisfactory for building a midwifery identity or for having midwives be ultimately accountable for their care.

## Conclusions

Despite these limitations, the projects have been an important developmental step within a country where midwives are unfamiliar as caregivers. Each of the projects has been accruing outcome data and reporting its results. This information is important in the evaluation of the projects and in the planning of midwifery care in other Canadian provinces. There are new projects in the formative stages whose developers look to the experience of the three pioneers. They hope to build on the existing projects and better anticipate many of their challenges. A cautionary point, however, is that unless planners clearly recognize the fundamental need for a legally defined midwifery role, they may create situations that will perpetuate the requirement for direct medical supervision.

Fortunately, there is new legislation in Ontario and Alberta, and legislative proposals are being developed in British Columbia, that will establish midwifery as an autonomous self-regulated profession. With these new legislative frameworks, the demonstration projects have a high potential for evolving from their present single-institution base to being a vital part of a network of midwifery services. The efforts to create and sustain the hospital demonstration projects could be no better rewarded.

REFERENCES

Barrington E 1985 Midwifery is catching. N C Press, Toronto
Buhler L, Glick N, Sheps S B 1988 Prenatal care: a comparative evaluation of nurse-midwives and family physicians. Canadian Medical Association Journal 139: 397–403
Burtch B 1992 The sociology of law: critical approaches to social control. Harcourt Brace Jovanovich, Toronto
Carty E, Effer S, Farquharson D, King J, Rice A, Tier D, Weatherston L, Wittmann B 1985 The Low-Risk Clinic: family care based on a midwifery model, 1981–1984. Shaughnessy Hospital Educational Services and the University of British Columbia School of Nursing, Vancouver, British Columbia

Flint C, Poulengeris P 1987 The 'Know Your Midwife' Report. Available from author, London

Grace Hospital Midwifery Program 1993 Statistics for the year ending 1992. Internal Grace Hospital unpublished report, Vancouver, British Columbia

Kaufman K, McDonald H 1988 A retrospective evaluation of a model of midwifery care. Birth 15(2): 95–99

McDonald H 1989 Intrapartum interventions: a comparative study of midwife and physician care. Unpublished master's thesis, McMaster University, Hamilton, Ontario, Canada

Martin E 1987 The woman in the body. Beacon Press, Boston

Rice A, Payne S, Mavis S 1993 Midwifery in a tertiary hospital setting: a Canadian experience. Proceedings of the 23rd International Congress of the International Confederation of Midwives. Vancouver, British Columbia

Torrance G M 1987 Socio-historical overview: the development of the Canadian health system. In: Coburn D, D'Arcy C, Torrance G M, New P (eds) Health and Canadian society. Fitzhenry & Whiteside, Markham, Ontario, p 6–35

# 11

# Midwifery practice in New Zealand: a dynamic discipline

*Judy Hedwig   Valerie Fleming*

## INTRODUCTION

The practice of midwifery in New Zealand is facing many challenges at the present time. Only 10 years ago the future for midwifery looked bleak, with the continuing medicalisation of childbirth and the attempts by some powerful nurse educators to deregister midwifery, downgrading it to a post-registration nursing programme. Midwifery has overcome these immense obstacles, however, to become a discipline, independent of both medicine and nursing.

However, the health services in New Zealand are currently undergoing radical changes, with the demise of 'free' hospital care having begun in early 1992. The emphasis of the health sector is now on profit with hospitals which are seen to be viable, to be turned into Crown Health Enterprises in mid-1993.

The future for midwifery is again uncertain, as while secondary care services are planned, the funding for primary care services has yet to be determined. Independent midwives may have to tender for their share of bulk funds, or join forces to have a voice. In such a climate of uncertainty, therefore, it is difficult to posit a model or even several models for midwifery practice.

This chapter, therefore, begins by describing a research-based model for midwifery practice which was developed in 1990. The process of developing the model is described in the hope that it may inspire other midwives to follow its decision trail and consider their own beliefs about practice. Limitations of the model are outlined, and an attempt to 'capture' present day influences on midwifery education and practice is then made. Finally some challenges are offered to midwives in clinical practice.

## A MODEL FOR MIDWIFERY PRACTICE IN NEW ZEALAND

### Use of models

According to Wilson (1985) a model:

represents some aspect of reality, concrete or abstract, by means of a likeness which may be structural, pictorial, diagrammatic or mathematical. A model, unlike a theory, does not focus on the relationships among phenomena but rather on their structure or function. A model is essentially an analogy, a symbolic representation of an idea.

Galt & Smith (1976) describe a model as:

a mental construct which is a unit in a body of theory and which aids the social scientist in conceptualising and generalising aspects of social behaviour or processes through the device of subtracting detail and generalising from specifics.

Benner (1984) also states that formal models provide a model of reality, an abstract representation like a map. Models, therefore, have been widely used in disciplines such as nursing and medicine to outline the parameters of practice.

A model for midwifery practice can be seen as valuable for the following reasons. It can be used to:

- integrate complex data
- act as an aid in communication:
  —between midwives and their employers
  —for educators organising their study programmes
  —for midwives communicating with their clients and colleagues
- clarify who the midwives are, and what midwives do, want, and need for:
  —developing their profession
  —educating trainee midwives
  —communicating with employers and clients.

# Development of a research-based model for midwifery practice

A qualitative study by Hedwig (1990) adapted these ideas to develop a model for midwifery practice in New Zealand. Data were obtained from 25 recently qualified midwives in practice in hospitals throughout the country. As midwifery was facing many challenges, it was seen to be imperative that the views of midwives were considered when planning changes in the educational and practice settings of midwives in New Zealand.

Two focusing research questions were used to guide Hedwig's study in the areas of midwifery education and practice.

1. How was their polytechnic education perceived by the recently qualified midwives?
2. What organisational and professional factors are perceived by the midwives as being present in the workplace that encourage them to remain practising within the profession?

The initial results indicated the following needs for midwives: flexible training requirements; realisation of their prior nursing experiences; continuing professional educational needs, and expansion of practical experiences to contribute to the development of a growing autonomous midwifery practice. Hedwig (1990) therefore proposed an initial model for midwifery practice (Fig. 11.1) which was offered to help clarify and integrate aspects of complex and varied issues.

This model of midwifery practice, which is a 'building' model or a 'model-in-process', arose out of the newly qualified midwives' perceptions of their education and employment. To explain the model requires an understanding of the outer parameters as well as the progression of the midwife within the circle of practice. The outer framework represents environmental, societal and cultural influences which encompass and impact on the midwife's working relationship with the woman.

Within this circle a linear progression takes place after completion of midwifery education and when the midwife enters practice (phase one). The linear phases which will be discussed in more detail below involve a progression through needs (phase two), practice goals (phase three) and job satisfaction (phase four). This linear progression must always be seen as taking place within the parameters of the outer circle.

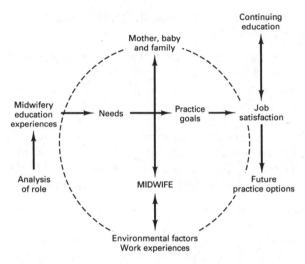

**Figure 11.1** An initial model for midwifery practice.

## Phase 1: entering practice

The first phase began as the newly registered midwife enters the practice environment and became aware of the strengths and limitations of her midwifery education, including her clinical experiences. This phase was described as covering the first 6 weeks of practice in any midwifery area.

## Phase 2: needs

After the first 6 weeks, certain ongoing needs were identified by the midwives as requiring to be met, so enabling the midwife to move through to the next phase. These included the following:

**1. Knowledge needs.** The midwives surveyed expressed a need for greater knowledge. They stressed the importance of continually updating their education both through long-term attendance at university, and by attending staff development in hospital programmes. Midwifery skill workshops which are available at various polytechnics and through different New Zealand College of Midwives regional group educational meetings were also seen as a source of furthering midwifery knowledge.

**2. Peer support needs.** The midwives saw the importance of having midwifery peer support to share, discuss and develop new ideas, knowledge, trends and changes. They especially mentioned that they liked networking with and having the comradeship of other midwives. They saw the recently established professional College of Midwives as a forum for expressing the views of practising midwives and providing a partnership between midwives and consumers.

**3. Personal needs.** The research showed that some newly qualified midwives in New Zealand are older, more mature and have more life experiences. These include having had children, or a wide variety of professional experiences, such as working in different areas within hospital or community settings. This maturity and experience needs acknowledgement in the work environment.

**4. Interpersonal needs.** These were largely defined as involving recognition as a professional and encompassed the following requirements:

• An orientation programme and a mentor when starting a new job even if it was a return to an area previously worked in. This would enable socialisation into the new position and work place.

• To be accepted and recognised as an educated and skilled practitioner by colleagues, doctors and clients.

• To have control and power over certain situations, including medical acceptance of the midwife's expertise in various situations, such as emergencies.

• To have support not only from people the midwife works with, but also from management.

• To work harmoniously with other staff in order to achieve a happy atmosphere for the women in their care.

• To have more flexibility within the system especially from older practising midwives who have been in their positions for a long time. Flexibility of the hours of work/shifts/time-in-lieu and flexibility of the delivery of care given to the women, e.g. more involvement with community-based schemes, was mentioned.

**5. Self needs.** The midwives identified the need for certain levels of experience, confidence and assertiveness that they considered were essential for competent practice.

The above five needs represent the second phase, and have to be addressed if the midwife is to feel strong and confident enough to support the women for whom she is caring. There are similarities between this phase and Benner's (1984) third and fourth stages of competence and proficiency in levels of expertise of the provider.

*Phase 3: practice goals*

Whereas phase two focused on the needs of the beginning practitioner, this third phase of the model encompassed three types of practice goals or achievements, relating to ongoing professional development.

**1. Personal goals.** These were described as perceptual and included working within a personal philosophy of wellness and the promotion of women's health. They included the ability to say 'I am a midwife' and know what that means for self and women.

**2. Self-focused goals.** These are:

- working as an autonomous practitioner
- being able to make decisions
- taking responsibility or being 'in charge' of situations.

These goals arose within the organisational context of midwifery. They were also coupled with the midwife's perception of her role in research, and her continual self-evaluation of where she is and what she is doing in order to provide a high standard of care. These goals included continuing education and self development programmes.

**3. Client-focused goals.** The midwives loved working with mothers and babies and enjoyed working alongside women in labour. They were culturally sensitive to all groups that they worked with, especially the Maori women and their 'whanau'. (The Maori word 'whanau' means 'to be born' or 'bear a child' but is used as a wider concept to illustrate an extended close-knit family.) They did not like fragmentation of care, preferring the idea of a continuity of care scheme where they could care for woman throughout her pregnancy, confinement and postnatal phase. They enjoyed the situation where they could help the woman or couple, and where they had the ability and confidence to empower women to question and ask for alternative choices.

The level to which these three types of goals were achieved was associated with the extent to which needs are met in the earlier phase.

*Phase 4: job satisfaction*

As the practice goals of Phase 3 are achieved, the midwife moves on to the fourth phase of the model, encompassing job satisfaction and, presumably, increased likelihood of remaining in the midwifery workplace. Job satisfaction arose from organisational, personal and professional factors and included:

- personal satisfaction derived from autonomy of practice
- maintaining one's own self-esteem by taking responsibility
- leaving work feeling 'I have achieved something'
- getting positive reinforcement and feedback from clients and colleagues.

This phase was closely linked to the first three phases and represents the achievement of these.

## Ongoing development of the model

If they are to be useful, models need regular review. The above phases have focused on the midwife in practice. A component within midwifery which was identified as needing further development, was the analysis of the role of the practising midwife for her own educational purposes and for developing ongoing aims for education and practice. This would serve two purposes:

1. provide continuing educational and skill workshops to keep the practising midwife up to date with current trends, and
2. feedback into the initial education of the midwife.

Consumer groups could also play an important role in this analysis by communicating their needs to the midwife.

Models however, are limiting in that they are 'frozen', simplistic versions of a reality which is actually fluid, dynamic and multidimensional (Belenky et al 1986).

Rather than update the model, therefore, we have chosen for the remainder of the chapter to discuss some of the complex network of forces which now influence midwifery education and practice in New Zealand.

## MIDWIFERY EDUCATION

Entry to midwifery practice can only come after a prescribed course of education, culminating in a state examination, has been successfully completed. A brief historical overview shows the changing focus of midwifery education throughout this century, in New Zealand.

The registration of midwives came about in New Zealand in

1904. Prior to this, there had been little control over entry to midwifery practice, most midwives having apprenticed themselves to an experienced midwife and learned their skills from her. The 1904 Act required all midwives to be registered; to do this, either a formal education in midwifery (class A midwives) was needed, or references of support from a medical practitioner (class B midwives) were obtained (Mein-Smith 1986).

Midwifery education involved a course of 6 months at a recognised training school for those who were already registered nurses, and for a longer period for 'direct entry' midwives. Although the respective training periods were to change over the years and direct entry midwifery was to follow on from maternity nurse training in the 1920s, these two educational routes for entry to midwifery practice remained in place for many years. However, from 1957, when 'obstetric nursing' was incorporated into the general nursing curriculum, the popularity of direct entry midwifery had declined. Midwifery thus became a post-registration certificate for nurses, essential for promotion in any clinical area, with direct entry courses being phased out in the 1970s.

Nursing education also underwent major changes in the 1970s. The New Zealand Government of the time was very concerned about the current system of nursing. There was a high 'drop out' rate of nurses undertaking the hospital-based training programmes, together with a shortage of qualified nursing tutors and a lack of retention of nursing staff. Consequently the Government asked the World Health Organization to provide a nurse consultant to look into this. Dr Helen Carpenter, a qualified nurse from the University of Toronto, with extensive experience, including a PhD in maternal and child health was brought to New Zealand on a short-term contract as a consultant. At that time she was the Director of the School of Nursing at the University of Toronto, Canada.

Dr Carpenter's report recommended that all hospital school of nursing programs leading to registration as nurses be discontinued (Carpenter 1971). In their place, programs which focused on educational goals rather than service needs were to be implemented in tertiary education institutions. Midwifery education, as a post-registration nursing program was also to make this change. Midwifery was now seen from the perspective of medical science, technology and education, thereby placing it in the hands of two masters, the obstetric profession and educational institutions.

Midwifery education was first offered through the polytechnics in 1980, as one option of the Advanced Diploma of Nursing (ADN). To be accepted for this programme 2 years' experience as a registered nurse was required, at least one of which was to be spent in the area of speciality. The number of places for student midwives on the programmes was determined by individual polytechnics, who had to balance midwifery with nurses seeking advanced certification in such areas as medical, surgical, psychiatric or community nursing. Combined with this, the difficulty that the student midwives had in attempting to fulfil the prerequisites of the Advanced Diploma of Nursing, as well as the Nursing Council's requirements for registration as a midwife, led to a huge drop in the numbers of graduating midwives.

Nursing Council statistics show that in the mid-1970s graduating midwives numbered between 155 and 165 per year. Only 120 midwives registered in 1980; these figures reflected midwives who registered from the last hospital-based programmes and the first run by polytechnics. The main shock was to come the following year when only 18 New Zealand-educated midwives were admitted to the register. Such low numbers were to remain the norm for almost the next decade, reaching a low in 1982 of 13. In 1985, only 18.75% (27) midwives who registered in New Zealand had been educated in local programs (Nursing Council 1986). The remainder, who were recruited to fill the gaps, had mostly trained in Australian and United Kingdom midwifery programs.

The Advanced Diploma of Nursing (including the midwifery option) was evaluated in 1984/1985. Detailed questionnaires were sent out to all 698 graduates from the Advanced Diploma of Nursing courses since 1979 as well as to 149 supervisors or senior colleagues who could comment on 'on the job performance'. A total of 574 and 131 were returned respectively. It was evident from this evaluation that neither the midwives who graduated from joint midwifery/advanced diploma programmes nor their service providers were fully satisfied with midwifery education. (Kennedy & Taylor 1987). A total of 60% of the graduates from the midwifery courses made suggestions for change, most of which were also recommended by the senior nursing personnel. Kennedy & Taylor (1987) reported that two options were generally favoured by those surveyed:

1. that the midwifery for registration option be separated from the ADN courses, or
2. that the midwifery option remain within the ADN courses but extensive modifications be made.

On the recommendation of this report, urgent changes were made and in 1989 the first 'stand-alone' programs leading to midwifery registration were offered at Auckland, Wellington and Dunedin. It was not until 1992 that two more polytechnics, Waikato and Christchurch introduced similar stand-alone programs.

By this time direct entry midwifery was also being offered from two polytechnics. Each of these programs was of 3 years' duration, the Auckland program being offered as a diploma and Otago's providing New Zealand's first degree in midwifery. These programs have only been funded as pilots for 4 years and are being closely monitored by the Nursing Council of New Zealand and the New Zealand Qualification's Authority.

Concerning the Otago program, applications for admission with credits from registered midwives who wish to obtain a degree in midwifery, are currently being considered. These developments are exciting for midwifery in New Zealand and in the future will lead to the creation of master's degrees in midwifery.

Although no university has yet taken up the challenge of offering papers in midwifery in this country, it is possible that some time in the near future the polytechnics and universities will work together to form a coordinated program from diploma level through to master's degrees.

## MIDWIFERY PRACTICE

In August 1990, section 54 of the Nurses' Act 1977 was amended by government, to allow midwives in New Zealand to take responsibility for the care of a woman throughout her pregnancy, labour and postnatal period, which since 1971 had been solely the role of the medical practitioners. The then Minister of Health, Helen Clark, hailed the passing of the legislation as offering 'greater choice in childbirth services to pregnant woman and their families' (Department of Health 1990).

New Zealand midwives practising at the time of writing (1992) therefore, have had opportunities to practise autonomously for 2 years. The College of Midwives has been working to ensure the success of autonomous practice. Midwives have chosen to practise in a number of ways, all of which are women-centred. Midwives recognise that, while they are prepared to practise without medical input, many women still wish their general practitioner or a consultant obstetrician be involved in their pregnancy, labour and birth. However, the relationship between midwives and medical practitioners has changed to one of collegiality rather than a supervisory role.

Whether independently or in partnership with a nominated medical practitioner, midwives are now providing a continuity of care for women which, until the Nurses' Amendment Act 1990, was practically nonexistent, except in the case of a few domiciliary midwives who received poor remuneration for their efforts. Throughout the country, midwives are now offering complete or shared prenatal care. This is a great step forward, as women who are pregnant today still generally follow a structured process through the prenatal period, beginning with the diagnosing of a pregnancy and continuing with the monitoring and treatment of that pregnancy. The monitoring consists of regular visits where blood tests, weighing, urine and blood pressure testing are performed. A ritual described by Byatt (1985) as taking place in the 1950s can still be seen today in some institutions. Indeed, the introduction over the last decade of 'routine' ultrasound scans has intensified this ritual further, and it now appears that women's dates cannot be relied upon.

Such an approach represents the immense control of the medical profession over women. It is an approach which has also been harnessed by many nurses and midwives. This control is extremely well organised, almost from the moment of conception. However, with the advent of autonomous midwifery practice, it is an approach which is being challenged both by women and midwives. The focus by midwives is now on developing a rapport with each woman and ascertaining her needs and wishes. Prenatal visits are not always so frequent and are often carried out in a woman's home, even if she has elected to have her baby in hospital.

Midwives also offer a number of options for women during the birthing process. Autonomous midwifery practice permits midwives to attend births at home, in birthing units or in hospitals. The place of birth is explored with the woman, and the people who support her prior to the time of birth and, if a hospital birth is chosen, the expected length of stay is also discussed.

## THE THEORETICAL BASIS FOR MIDWIFERY PRACTICE TODAY

Like nursing some 20 or 30 years ago, midwifery in New Zealand and elsewhere today, is suffering from the lack of a theoretical framework on which to base its practice. In this period, many nurse scholars have developed nursing theories, several of which now form the basis for both nursing education and nursing practice. This is not to say that individual nurses, practising alongside midwives, work to a theoretical framework, while midwives do not.

Such has been the dominance of the medical profession in this area, that alternatives are only just beginning to be considered. Bryar (1988) bemoans the lack of conceptual frameworks in midwifery practice and suggests, as an alternative, a variation on the 'nursing process'. However, the nursing process has developed from a reductionist approach to science which breaks down concepts into their constituent parts. It is therefore a similar approach to that of medical science, and its suitability for midwifery and nursing practice in the area of birthing must be questioned.

Given the wishes of midwives and women to have a service in which the personal nature of experience is acknowledged, some of the nursing theories which have developed from a humanistic framework may be more relevant, such as Paterson & Zderad's (1976) theory, which derives from existential phenomenology and focuses on the interaction between nurse and client. Other humanistic nursing theories which could form a basis for practice in this area are those of Rogers (1970) and Parse (1981).

As midwifery in New Zealand begins to move away from the medical model, midwives are simultaneously seeking independence from the nursing profession. The suitability of nursing theories as a basis for midwifery practice is thus brought into question. While nursing has not specifically aligned itself with the feminist movement (Speedy 1987), the counter-hegemonic struggle in New Zealand, resulting from the alliance between consumers and midwives described above, owes much to the feminist crusade. Feminist theory as a basis for midwifery practice is briefly explored below.

Speedy (1987) presents a thought-provoking article on the relationship of feminism and nursing which may also be relevant for midwifery. It is worth considering midwifery practice in relation to each of the four 'mainstream' feminist theories: liberal feminism, Marxist feminism, radical feminism and socialist feminism. The New Zealand College of Midwives has stated categorically that midwifery is a feminist profession, and its recent history would ratify this belief. However, there are some midwives who would not consider themselves feminists, so the adoption of such an approach must be tempered with caution.

The issue of theory-based practice is immense, and leaves many unanswered questions. The challenge may be for midwives in New Zealand to develop and test their own theories, and once again lead the world in developments in midwifery. However, the partnership with women which has been promoted by the New Zealand College of Midwives must remain paramount.

## CHALLENGES TO MIDWIFERY PRACTICE

The proposed model for midwifery practice which was presented at the beginning of this chapter, was created out the research undertaken before the Nurses' Amendment Act 1990 was passed, so the model was not used or validated. It was, however, tested and adopted by a group of midwives who have been advocating changes to the present midwifery education programs and the pilot direct entry midwifery programs. These midwives have stated that there have been more opportunities, over the past 2 years, in their workplaces: to extend their knowledge through ongoing educational programs, to be effective patient advocates for women and to practice midwifery autonomously in a variety of settings.

While we have not proposed a further model, we have discussed, the necessity for a theoretical framework for midwifery practice. Each midwife has her own framework or model which underlies her midwifery practice. This framework will comprise her own beliefs and values about midwifery and will have developed through her education, practice and life experiences.

Midwives in New Zealand are leaders in terms of their rejection of the medical model of obstetric practice, their independence and their woman-centred approach. They now need to take stock of where they are with their own framework of midwifery practice by enhancing, developing and building upon it. These are the challenges for midwives within our country today.

REFERENCES

Belenky M S, Clinchy B M, Goldberger N R, Tarule J M 1986 Womens ways of knowing: the development of self, voice, and mind. Basic Books, USA

Benner P 1984 From novice to expert: excellence and power in clinical nursing practice. Addison-Wesley, California

Bryar R 1988 Midwifery and models of care. Midwifery 4: 111–117

Byatt A S 1985 Still life. Penguin London

Carpenter H 1971 An improved system of nursing education in New Zealand. Department of Health, Wellington, New Zealand

Department of Health 1990 Nurses' Amendment Act 1990: Information for health care providers. Government Printers, Wellington, New Zealand

Galt A, Smith L 1976 Models and the study of social change. John Wiley, New York

Hedwig J A 1990 Midwives: preparation and practice. Master of Arts thesis, Massey University, Palmerston North, New Zealand

Kennedy S, Taylor A 1987 An evaluation of Advanced Diploma in Nursing courses. Department of Education, Wellington, New Zealand

Mein-Smith P 1986 Maternity in dispute: New Zealand 1920–1935. Government Printers, Wellington, New Zealand

Nursing Council of New Zealand 1986 Annual workforce statistics. Unpublished

Parse R R 1981 Man-living-health: a theory of nursing. John Wiley, New York

Paterson J G, Zderad L T 1976 Humanistic nursing. John Wiley, New York

Rogers M E 1970 An introduction to the theoretical basis of nursing. F A Davis, Philadelphia

Speedy S 1987 Feminism and the professionalisation of nursing. Australian Journal of Advanced Nursing 42: 20–28

Wilson H 1985 Research in nursing. Addison-Wesley, California

# Related issues

# 12

# The impact of human immunodeficiency virus infection on midwifery

*Sheelagh Scattergood*

## INTRODUCTION

When the problem of infection with human immunodeficiency virus (HIV) first made the headlines, the reaction by midwives mirrored the reaction of the population at large. This was a previously unrecognised infection which affected quite specific groups within society but was not of any great consequence to individuals outside those specific groups. Gradually it became obvious that the early view of the limits of this infection was a false one. By the early 1990s, some 10 years since the initial information about HIV, it has been described as 'a pandemic out of control. It is dynamic, volatile and unstable and, more importantly, the major impact is yet to come (Mann 1992).

# The nature of the problem

The human immunodeficiency virus belongs to a group of viruses known as retroviruses which are characterised by the production of a specific viral enzyme, reverse transcriptase. The enzyme is used to transcribe the genetic codes of the virus from RNA to the DNA of the host cells by a retrograde step. The enzyme is very important in the identification process, and may also be the key to the development of a means of controlling replication of the virus. Some of the drugs currently used in HIV management are inhibitors of reverse transcriptase.

The structure of the virus is complex (Fig. 12.1) The outer layer is lipid structure with glycoproteins embedded in it. These are designated GP120 and GP41. Within this lies a protein shell made up of protein antigens designated P24 and P18. These antigens, or their antibodies, are also used in the diagnostic tests for HIV infection. This protein shell encloses the virion which is the central part of the virus and contains the RNA.

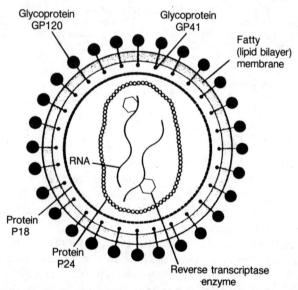

**Figure 12.1**  Schematic diagram of the HIV virus (English National Board 1987). (Figures 12.1 and 12.2 are reproduced, by kind permission of the ENB, from the learning package *AIDS: Meeting the Challenge*. The second edition is available under the title *Caring for people with sexually transmitted diseases including HIV disease*. ENB 1994)

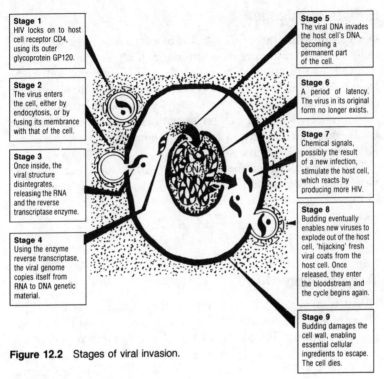

**Stage 1**
HIV locks on to host cell receptor CD4, using its outer glycoprotein GP120.

**Stage 2**
The virus enters the cell, either by endocytosis, or by fusing its membrane with that of the cell.

**Stage 3**
Once inside, the viral structure disintegrates, releasing the RNA and the reverse transcriptase enzyme.

**Stage 4**
Using the enzyme reverse transcriptase, the viral genome copies itself from RNA to DNA genetic material.

**Stage 5**
The viral DNA invades the host cell's DNA, becoming a permanent part of the cell.

**Stage 6**
A period of latency. The virus in its original form no longer exists.

**Stage 7**
Chemical signals, possibly the result of a new infection, stimulate the host cell, which reacts by producing more HIV.

**Stage 8**
Budding eventually enables new viruses to explode out of the host cell, 'hijacking' fresh viral coats from the host cell. Once released, they enter the bloodstream and the cycle begins again.

**Stage 9**
Budding damages the cell wall, enabling essential cellular ingredients to escape. The cell dies.

**Figure 12.2**   Stages of viral invasion.

## Infection with HIV

When infection occurs (Fig. 12.2) the glycoproteins, GP120 and GP41, of the outer lipid layer of the virus bind to the receptor sites on the outer membrane of the host cells. HIV has a high affinity for certain host cells including some cells of the central nervous system and CD4 helper cells. The latter cells play an important role in the immune system of the host. The virus then transcribes its own RNA into the DNA of the host cell using the specific enzyme. Viral DNA is then replicated with every division of the affected cells.

The virus, then, undergoes a period of latency. During this period, paradoxically, the virus continues to be replicated at each division of the infected cell and it is still able to infect new cells in the host. Eventually the virus becomes active again and the host DNA produces viral RNA. In addition, new enzymes and viral proteins are produced to form new virions. Finally the host cell dies and the new virus particles escape to invade other host cells.

## Effects of infection

Once a large number of CD4 cells are infected or destroyed both cell-mediated immunity and antibody formation are severely reduced. At this stage the body is in a state of immune deficiency for the control of new infections or developing tumours. The host system can still respond to previously encountered infections but not to new ones. Neonates infected with HIV at or before birth are unable to establish any immunity systems before the invading HIV destroys the ability to do so.

The virus belongs to the subfamily *Lentivirinae*. There are two viruses identified so far, within this subgroup, which are known to infect humans.

- HIV-1: the more common virus worldwide
- HIV-2: mostly confined to West Africa.


## Transmission of HIV

HIV is transmitted both laterally and longitudinally (Table 12.1). There is a delay between infection and the time when detection is possible. During this biological time lag the infected people are asymtomatic and do not consider themselves at risk or as being a risk to others. The time lag is very variable. It can be less than 6 months but time lags of up to 42 months have been recorded. The HIV has been shown to affect many organs directly or indirectly. These include the brain, heart, gastrointestinal tract and bone marrow, in addition to the lymphocytes.

The US Centers for Disease Control have proposed a classification system based on the known progression of the disease. This progression takes the following format:

**Table 12.1** The means of transmission of HIV

| | |
|---|---|
| Laterally | Sexual contact, or<br>Exchange of blood and body fluids by:<br>    Injecting drug use<br>    Transfusion of blood or blood products |
| Longitudinally | Mother to infant:<br>    Across the placenta<br>    During the birth process<br>    By breast feeding |

1.  Seronegative but infected
2.  Seropositive but symptom-free
3.  Subclinical immune deficiency
4.  AIDS-related complex (ARC)
5.  AIDS or the full acquired immune deficiency syndrome

It is still too early in the study of this disease to known if this route of progression is always followed.

The estimated mean time between infection and the development of full-blown AIDS is 5.5 years but up to 14 years have been recorded. The majority of known infected women worldwide are in the seropositive but symptom-free group (Mann 1992).

## THE EXTENT OF THE PROBLEM

### The global view

Today the AIDS pandemic is out of control. Its course through and within global society has not been affected in any substantial manner by the actions taken thus far at the national or international level (Mann 1992). Since the first AIDS cases were reported the pandemic has swept the world. In 1980 an estimated 100 000 people worldwide were infected with HIV. Today the estimated number is 12 million adults throughout the world and it is recognised that this is a conservative estimate. There are:

*   7 000 000 in Africa
*   1 000 000 in America
*   1 000 000 in Asia
*   500 000 in Europe.

Of these millions, seven are male and over four million are female. The ratio of women to men is increasing. There is a danger that reading such large figures induces a certain numbness as if the noughts really do mean nothing.

The AIDS pandemic has been described as being dynamic, volatile and unstable.

### Dynamic

The pandemic is dynamic in that it has continued to spread in the countries that were first identified as having a problem. For example, it has been predicted that in the 3 years (1992–1995) between 120 000 and 240 000 infections will occur in the USA and that in 1991 750 000 new infections occurred in Europe (Mann 1992).

The incidence in developing countries is also increasing rapidly; for instance the rate of HIV seropositive pregnant women in Nairobi was 2% in 1985 but 13% in 1991. There has not been any country where HIV has been recognised and then transmission has ceased. In addition to the continued spread in these countries, the virus has travelled to other countries which had not previously recorded infection, for example, parts of rural Africa, Greenland, Paraguay and various Pacific islands (Mann 1992).

*Volatile*

The pandemic is volatile or changeable. The rate and method of spread in different countries varies. For example, the epidemic in Thailand has become 10 times larger (on a population basis) than the spread in the UK. In India, the spread is mostly heterosexual and increasing very rapidly. By 1995 it is estimated that the number of infected Asians will exceed the total number of infected people in all the industralised countries. It is only a matter of time before all communities have the virus among their people.

*Unstable*

The pandemic is also unstable and evolving, in that different types of people are becoming infected. Whereas in the early days, midwives might have had little involvement, now they are increasingly caring for infected clients. Although this infection was first recognised among homosexual men, today the HIV spreads throughout all parts of the community by all available routes. The chief route of infection is by that very common human activity, sexual intercourse. The first figures in 1981 in USA showed 97% of people with AIDS were male, and came from only two states. By 1990 this had changed to 11% being female 800 children were also affected, and the reports came from all 50 states.

The predictions for the pandemic is that the worst is yet to come. The figure released in 1992 estimated 500 000 people with AIDS worldwide (World Health Organization (WHO) 1992), but some very experienced workers regard this as excessively conservative and suggest a more realistic estimate would be 1.5 million adults and 500 000 children. As these figures are for AIDS, the number of HIV infections can only be guessed. The WHO projection that 30–40 million will be HIV infected by the year 2000 is also thought to be very conservative, but even so, from that (possibly very low) estimate at least 10 million adults and 5 million children can be expected to develop AIDS in the 1990s.

## The future in Europe

What will be the future of the epidemic in Europe? The early 1990s have seen an enormous upheaval in Europe. Following the collapse of the USSR there are civil wars, economic crises and social unrest in a number of countries. All these circumstances are likely to accelerate the spread of HIV.

## The UK position in 1994

In the UK homosexual groups reacted very positively to the situation and there are fewer cases of AIDS than had been predicted. The heterosexual spread, however, has been rising and this will have an ever-increasing effect on midwifery. The most recent figures for the UK (Figs 12.3 and 12.4) demonstrate the faster rate of increase in heterosexuals compared with the spread among homosexuals, even though the overall numbers of hetero-sexuals with HIV/AIDS is lower for the time being (Table 12.2).

The UK position in January 1994 was that 141 new cases of AIDS were reported. The *Communicable Disease Report* of February 1994 stated:

Of these 92 were probably infected through sexual intercourse between men, (12 died); 17 through sexual intercourse between men and women, (two died); eight through injecting drug use (two died); 11 through blood factor treatments (seven died) and eight through transmission from mother to infant (one died). The exposure categories of 7 cases (three died) were undetermined' (Public Health Laboratory Service 1994)

Since reporting began in 1982 to 30 September 1993 a total of 8115 AIDS cases (7496 male and 619 female) have been reported, of whom 5653 are known to have died. There was an increase in 11% (from 1307 to 1452) in the number of AIDS cases reported in the two 12-month periods from August 1990 to July 1992. The

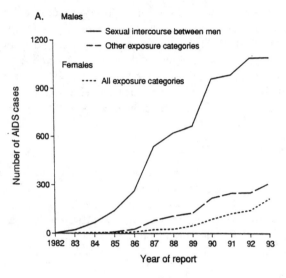

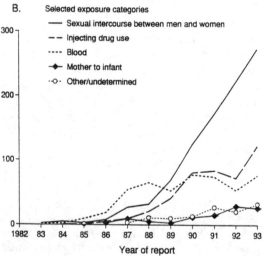

**Figure 12.3** AIDS cases in the United Kingdom to the end of December 1993: **A** sex, and and **B** exposure category by year of report. (Total = 8529 cases.)

number of cases attributed to sex between men increased by 10% (from 934 to 1026) over this period: the number of cases attributed to sex between men and women increased by 42% (150 to 213), and the number attributed to injecting drug use decreased

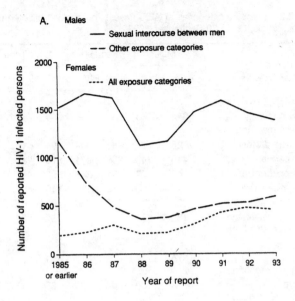

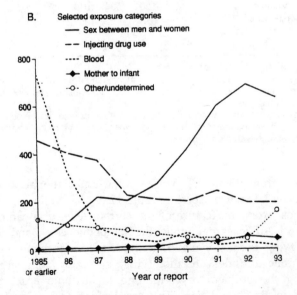

**Figure 12.4** Reported number of HIV-1 infected persons in the United Kingdom to the end of December 1993: **A** sex, and **B** exposure category by year of report. (Total = 21 015 reports, excluding 53 reports for which sex was not stated, and 33 reports for which year of report was not known.)

**Table 12.2** Exposure categories of AIDS cases, and of HIV-1 infected persons: cumulative totals, UK to 30 September 1993

| How the virus was probably acquired | Male AIDS | Male HIV-1 | Female AIDS | Female HIV-1 | Total AIDS | Total % | Total HIV-1[1] | Total % |
|---|---|---|---|---|---|---|---|---|
| Sexual intercourse | | | | | | | | |
| Between men | 6043 | 12475 | — | — | 6043 | 74 | 12475 | 61 |
| Between men and women | | | | | | | | |
| 'High risk' partner[2] | 26 | 71 | 68 | 344 | 94 | 1 | 415 | 2 |
| Other partner abroad[3] | 415 | 1143 | 258 | 971 | 673 | 8 | 2118 | 10 |
| Other partner UK | 43 | 77 | 34 | 142 | 77 | 1 | 219 | 1 |
| Under investigation | 7 | 118 | 3 | 131 | 10 | <1 | 249 | 1 |
| Injecting drug use (IDU) | 282 | 1704 | 122 | 760 | 404 | 5 | 2471 | 12 |
| IDU and sexual intercourse between men | 132 | 271 | — | — | 132 | 2 | 271 | 1 |
| Blood | | | | | | | | |
| Blood factor (e.g. haemophiliacs) | 375 | 1207 | 6 | 11 | 381 | 5 | 1218 | 6 |
| Blood/tissue transfer (e.g. transfusion) | 30 | 89 | 57 | 93 | 87 | 1 | 183 | 1 |
| Mother to infant | 46 | 100 | 53 | 101 | 99 | 1 | 202 | 1 |
| Other/undetermined | 97 | 615 | 18 | 120 | 115 | 1 | 769 | 4 |
| Total | 7496 | 17870 | 619 | 2673 | 8115 | 100 | 20590 | 100 |

[1] Includes 47 reports, sex not recorded.
[2] Includes men and women who had sex with infecting drug users, or with those infected through blood factor treatment or blood transfusion, and women who had sex with bisexual men.
[3] Includes persons without other identified risks from, or who have lived in, countries where the major route of HIV-1 transmission is through sexual intercourse between men and women.

by 25% (from 93 to 70). The regional and national variations within the UK can be seen in Table 12.3.

A most worrying feature of the current level of awareness of HIV and AIDS is that while the pandemic is expanding and intensifying, the national and international commitment is declining. Public attitudes are modifying, becoming complacent, or denying the problem or continuing to attribute it to defined groups in the population. The economic situation, which has resulted in increasing levels of unemployment and cuts in public spending, is creating a climate in which the infection can spread without control. There is less money available for major media

**Table 12.3** Geographical distribution and exposure category of HIV-1 infected persons: to end December 1993

| Country or region of first report | Sexual intercourse Between 'men'[1] | Between men (M) and women (F) M | F | NS² | Injecting drug use M | F | NS² | Blood | Other/ undetermined M | F | NS² | Cumulative 1984–Dec 93 |
|---|---|---|---|---|---|---|---|---|---|---|---|---|
| England | | | | | | | | | | | | |
| Northern | 194 | 33 | 25 | — | 44 | 12 | 1 | 88 | 9 | — | — | 406 |
| Yorkshire | 294 | 50 | 54 | — | 39 | 24 | — | 72 | 9 | 5 | — | 547 |
| Trent | 313 | 69 | 39 | 1 | 44 | 15 | — | 80 | 8 | 10 | — | 579 |
| E Anglia | 135 | 30 | 26 | — | 42 | 14 | — | 34 | 10 | 1 | — | 292 |
| NW Thames | 4757 | 241 | 336 | 5 | 282 | 127 | 2 | 56 | 193 | 62 | 12 | 6068 |
| NE Thames | 2626 | 347 | 409 | 1 | 174 | 114 | 1 | 183 | 235 | 55 | 19 | 4168 |
| SE Thames | 1591 | 185 | 234 | 1 | 169 | 78 | — | 134 | 58 | 31 | — | 2481 |
| SW Thames | 408 | 94 | 139 | — | 43 | 12 | — | 37 | 42 | 14 | 1 | 790 |
| Wessex | 302 | 33 | 33 | — | 27 | 8 | — | 38 | 11 | 7 | 1 | 460 |
| Oxford | 233 | 48 | 56 | 1 | 39 | 12 | 1 | 111 | 11 | 1 | 3 | 516 |
| S Western | 256 | 41 | 31 | — | 43 | 7 | — | 33 | 9 | 4 | — | 424 |
| W Midlands | 374 | 55 | 55 | — | 30 | 11 | — | 160 | 18 | 2 | — | 705 |
| Mersey | 129 | 14 | 14 | — | 10 | 9 | — | 43 | 14 | 1 | — | 234 |
| N Western | 610 | 63 | 38 | — | 50 | 29 | — | 120 | 11 | 3 | — | 924 |
| Wales | 184 | 42 | 26 | — | 10 | 2 | — | 56 | 13 | 2 | — | 335 |
| Northern Ireland | 63 | 11 | 14 | — | 3 | 3 | — | 20 | 2 | — | — | 116 |
| Scotland | 546 | 126 | 162 | — | 685 | 298 | 2 | 99 | 92 | 45 | 1 | 2056 |
| United Kingdom total | 13015 | 1482 | 1691 | 8 | 1734 | 775 | 7 | 1364 | 745 | 243 | 37 | 21101 |
| Channel Islands/Isle of Man | 15 | 1 | 2 | — | 4 | 3 | — | 3 | 2 | — | — | 30 |

[1] Includes 274 male drug users who also had sexual intercourse with other men.  ² Sex not stated on report.

activities to promote health education, information systems and free needle schemes for intravenous drug abusers. In spite of considerable hard work and enthusiasm in some areas, the overall trend is towards a feeling that the campaigners got it wrong. Because the pandemic has not yet touched the majority, or anyone they know personally, there is a developing opinion that its importance was greatly exaggerated.

The gap between the pandemic and the efforts to control it seemed to be narrowing in the late 1980s; whereas now it is widening rapidly. The 'safe sex' campaign for the use of condoms was challenged in the early 1990s because of the known failure rate of condoms as a contraceptive. As the failure rate in protection against a virus is not likely to be any better, the focus of the new health campaign is 'safer sex'. However, this is little consolation to those affected individuals for whom the impact is absolute, despite an overall condom failure rate of only 5%.

## HIV and women

The spread of HIV among women, and the consequences for unborn children as well as their mothers, reflects the status of women in many countries. It has been shown in Africa, for example, that women are becoming infected because they are unable to influence their husband's sexual behaviour. The women are monogamous but the men have many partners. It is no use preaching safer sex in these circumstances. Such situations are not confined to Africa. Many women in the UK do not have the social or economic power to influence the behaviour of their men folk. Midwives in the UK should not think that every one of the women in their care can insist on the use of condom.

The situation for women is serious. Not only may they be powerless to prevent the spread of infection, but also it is already suspected that progression from AIDS to death is more rapid in women. Most of the work on AIDS to date has been done with men; it may be that the effects on women are no different, but there is a need for further research before this hypothesis can be rejected.

Detection of HIV infection before the development of symptoms is not easy. Certain groups of women are at greater risk of the infection (see Table 12.4), and key infections may indicate that they also have the HIV. At present, however, the most common

**Table 12.4**  Groups of women at risk of HIV infection

All women who are sexually active but in particular:

   Intravenous drug users past and present

   Recipients of infected blood

   Those from countries with high infection rates e.g. Asia, sub-Saharan Africa

   Partners of haemophiliacs, bisexual males and injecting drug users

indicator of maternal disease is the development of symptoms in their infants.

## THE IMPACT TO DATE OF HIV ON MIDWIFERY

In the early years of this epidemic the impact of this new infection on midwifery was not very great. It was perceived that it affected very distinct groups in society and these were predominately male. It soon became obvious that women who were injecting drug users could also be affected. It was still thought that spread by heterosexual intercourse was unlikely because, it was argued, the structure of the vagina afforded protection for women. On the whole, it was only those centres where there were known drug abusers which saw early action to produce policies for the management of infected patients.

When the UK Government became concerned about the infection, a vigorous campaign was launched designed to enlighten the general public and make known the dangers of this new infection. Guidelines were produced for the management of infected patients by the health authorities. The information available at that time, the mid-1980s, was very limited. Neither the modes of transmission nor the fatal nature of the disease were fully understood, although it was recognised that babies could be infected in utero. As the knowledge of the virus developed, more precautions were advocated for health workers and it was recommended that special procedures should be drawn up for infected mothers.

The fact that these mothers were (and still are) mostly unidentified was to prove to be a major problem. In spite of the extensive health education campaign of the mid-1980s, most of the general public did not really understand the situation. Midwives were not much different, especially in areas where there were no known cases. A study undertaken in 1988 showed that of a one-in-five

**Table 12.5** Infection control measures to prevent transmission of blood-borne viruses in the health care setting (Department of Health 1991)

1. Apply good basic hygiene practices with regular hand washing.

2. Cover existing wounds or skin lesions with waterproof dressings.

3. Avoid invasive procedures if suffering from chronic skin lesions on hands.

4. Avoid contamination of person by appropriate use of protective clothing.

5. Protect mucous membranes of eyes, mouth and nose from blood splashes.

6. Prevent puncture wound, cuts and abrasions in the presence of blood.

7. Avoid sharps usage wherever possible.

8. Institute safe procedures for handling and disposal of needles and other sharps.

9. Institute approved procedures for sterilization and disinfection of instruments and equipment.

10. Clear up spillages of blood and other body fluids promptly and disinfect surfaces.

11. Institute a procedure for the safe disposal of contaminated waste.

sample of all community midwives in Scotland ($n = 272$) only 1.8% had experience with AIDS patients (Tierney et al 1990). Most midwives have not had to confront a life-threatening condition in their working lives, so many of them found it difficult to grasp the significance of the policies for prevention of infection. In an informal survey undertaken in 1992 in one city hospital (which serves a considerable community of drug abusers) not one midwife admitted to using eye protection against cord blood spurts or liquor splashes at delivery in spite of the fact that a form of eye protection was available in the delivery rooms (Scattergood 1992).

In spite of the lethargy of the public, midwives must become ever more vigilant as the number of infected mothers and babies rises. The main thrust of the guidelines issued by the Department of Health (1991) is that good practices are the best protection (Table 12.5).

## HIV testing

The issue of testing for HIV status is a very complex one, both in terms of the nature of the virus and the extent of the spread. The media reaction in the UK to the epidemic in the early 1980s has left a legacy of misinformation, mistrust, suspicion and stigma associated with the disease, all of which have complicated an already difficult situation. It is not easy to suggest to women that they should consider being tested; nor can it be easy for them to seek testing. The biological time lag means that there are infected individuals who cannot be identified. Those who have been tested and are seropositive can remain symptom-free without giving any clue to their infected state.

The heterosexual spread is through all levels of society and is not isolated to a defined group or groups. Although to date there are a greater number of men than women infected, the ratio of infected women to men is increasing.

So who should be tested? Given the reaction of the public to known seropositive individuals and the discriminatory actions of insurance companies and potential employers, it is unlikely that testing can be made compulsory. Some women present for voluntary testing if they feel themselves to be at risk. Others are offered the test if they come from a high risk group. The decision to request or accept testing can be a difficult one, even before having to face the results of the test. Anonymous testing is being carried out by the Department of Health in an attempt to assess the dimensions of the problem.

If a decision to be tested has been made, the results cannot always be presented in a clear-cut fashion. Positive results will be difficult to accept and will require support and counselling from the midwife and other agencies. A negative result may not be conclusive because of the biological time lag. If not explained properly, this can lead to a false sense of security. The need for retesting is another source of anxiety for the women. The early results from anonymous antenatal testing so far indicate a seropositive rate of 1 in 16 000 throughout the UK, but it is 1 in 500 in inner London; the range is from 1 in 200 to 1 in 1000 in some clinics (Ades et al 1991).

## THE ROLE OF THE MIDWIFE

### The need for counselling

There are aspects of the midwife's role which will change, and which in fact are already changing as the need arises. One of these is counselling. It has long been recognised that a part of the role of the midwife is that of counsellor, yet the available training and preparation for this skill is very variable. There is and will be an increasing demand for expertise in counselling to deal with the range of problems presented to midwives by the HIV infection.

In the 1990s, our knowledge of HIV is that the infection leads inevitably to death and our management is limited. As the only known variable is the length of time between infection and death, women are faced with 'when' rather than 'if'. Seropositive mothers will have to face the knowledge of a reduced life expectancy which may be months or maybe years. There are other issues to be discussed before embarking on testing for HIV status, such as uncertainty about the partner's HIV status and the health of present or future children.

Midwives need to be aware of a range of emotions associated with a positive HIV status. The mother may feel guilty for putting her child at risk and may have to face a very traumatic decision as to whether she should seek a termination of the pregnancy. Midwives will require all the interpersonal skills they can muster to be able to support the mother through this difficult time. This may include an awareness of lay groups which offer long-term support and counselling, such as Positively Women. Midwives will need to develop their own strategies for coping with the whole range of human emotions and may even find the mothers have directed their anger towards them. The midwives themselves will require support from their colleagues so that they can offer mothers the care they require.

## ANTEPARTUM CARE

Among pregnant women with symptomatic HIV disease there is an increased incidence of complications. In one study, all the pregnancies were complicated by low birth weight, prematurity, fetal deaths in utero or stillbirth (Koonin et al 1989). Many of these women were already at risk from their lifestyles which included drug abuse, smoking, poor nutrition and little antenatal care. As well as these risk factors the results supported the assertion that as HIV infection progresses to AIDS the fetal and maternal outcomes are less favourable. Evidence from the USA indicates that the most common cause of death is pneumocystis carnii pneumonia (Koonin et al 1989).

Although the numbers are still low, especially in some parts of the country, midwives must be aware that any or many of the expectant women in their care may be infected. In the future, probably an increasing number will be aware of their status and will present at any stage of the progression of the HIV infection. In the early 1990s most women who are known to be infected, are symptom-free. For these women it is likely that pregnancy will not cause a deterioration in their condition and the HIV infection will not cause any increase in pregnancy-related problems. The major impact on these women will be the fear of the possible infection of the fetus.

At present the mother–infant transmission rate is estimated at 30% (Bastin et al 1992). This figure may be inaccurate as there are considerable difficulties in diagnosing the infection in the neonate. Babies may test seropositive in the early months because of maternal–fetal transmission of antibodies. Subsequent testing when the baby is older may produce a seronegative result.

Women who are already showing symptoms will require careful management to prevent a worsening of their condition, or to sustain them through an AIDS-related illness.

## Drug therapy in pregnancy

The main antiviral drugs belong to the dideoxynucleoside family, which inhibit the viral enzyme reverse transcriptase and thus can inhibit replication of the virus. AZT is the best known example of these drugs. It can be given after 14 weeks of pregnancy by which time organogensis is complete. It is known to cross the placental barrier and has been effective in preventing perinatal transmission in laboratory animals. The main side-effect, however, is suppression of the bone marrow, causing anaemia or thrombocytopenia. It may also affect the fetal marrow and can lead to intrauterine growth retardation (Nanda 1990).

Newer members of this drug family such as 2′, 3′-dideoxyinosine are less toxic to the bone marrow (Yarchoan et al 1989). Other drugs which may be used to complement AZT are designed to prevent infections such as pneumocystis pneumonia. Drugs such as trimethoprim and sulphamethoxazole are used prophylactically in this respect.

## Antenatal surveillance

HIV-infected women require increased surveillance in pregnancy, to monitor the HIV status and the development and wellbeing of the fetus. Regular fetal assessment by non-stress tests and serial ultrasound scans should be carried out for all known cases, even those who are asymptomatic. A sudden decline in immune status can lead to opportunistic infections which may prove fatal.

Other factors which complicate the issue, such as drug abuse or malnutrition, may also need assessment and active management.

Invasive procedures such as chorionic villus sampling and amniocentesis should be approached with caution and only undertaken after full consultation with the parents since such procedures may contaminate a non-infected fetus (Efantis & Sinclair 1990)

## Precautions for midwives in antepartum care

Antepartum care includes routine blood testing for all women. This procedure carries the risk of needle stick injuries and blood spillage. The routine wearing of gloves is recommended for the procedure of venepuncture, or for any procedure involving contact with blood or body fluids. Glove puncture rates as high as 48% have been recorded, so that some centres now advocate the use of double gloves (Kabukoba & Young 1992).

A recent study assessed the efficiency of minimising contamination of the skin of attendants at delivery with mother's body fluids (Kabukoba & Young 1992). It was reported that about half the practitioners and assistants at vaginal delivery had contaminated hands or arms or both. Of the staff investigated, 23% ($n = 226$) had broken skin, mostly on the hands and, in particular, in the nail beds. A worrying feature was that 35% of the total were not wearing gloves. This study was carried out in London which has the highest incidence of HIV infection in England and the report concluded that: 'the current practices for preventing contamination are inadequate and that staff may be at risk of contracting viral diseases while practising obstetrics'.

Any procedures which involve body fluids must therefore be carried out with much more attention to prevention of spread of the virus. Women who suffer antepartum haemorrhage or premature rupture of membranes are a particular infection risk.

As the point has already been made about the difficulty of knowing who is infected, it is especially important that the precautions to prevent the spread of infection should be universal. Routine precautions for all procedures for all women are essential, in order to safeguard not only the staff but also the women attending for maternity care.

The management of women known to be infected should require precautions which are no different, providing they are symptom-free.

## INTRAPARTUM CARE

Women with HIV infection are more likely to have increased blood loss than the uninfected; HIV infection is associated with a reduced thrombocyte count and they are therefore more at risk of haemorrhage, Midwives need to be aware of the possibility and particularly vigilant. The incidence of abruption of the placenta is higher in drug abusers and anaemia is common. This infection increases the effects of blood loss. For those women with the symptoms of HIV, there is an increased risk of complications such as premature labour and stillbirth.

In addition to the concerns about spreading infection from the women with HIV, there must be vigilance to reduce the risk of any other infections spreading to those who are immunocompromised. The relatively simple infections which cause mild distress or inconvenience to others, can prove fatal to those with AIDS-related complex (ARC) or AIDS (Table 12.6)

It cannot be assumed that all infants of women with HIV infection will become infected themselves. It must be a major concern to all midwives that their actions do not contribute to transmitting infection to a fetus who would otherwise not be infected. Procedures which penetrate the skin, such as the application of a fetal scalp electrode or fetal blood sampling, should never be undertaken lightly.

**Table 12.6** Key infections associated with HIV infection

Protracted herpes simplex

Extensive vaginal candidiasis

Aggressive cervical disease

Fulminating pelvic inflammatory disease

Accelerated syphilis infection

Cytomegalovirus

Toxoplasmosis

## Precautions for midwives during labour and delivery

The management of all women in labour should follow the normal patterns of care included in the guidelines for prevention of infection. These universal precautions should be what they aim to be: precautions which are universal. There should not be any let-up in their application, whenever a woman is in labour, be it in hospitals with known infected or high risk women, in hospitals with women who seem to be at low risk of HIV, or in the home.

The findings by Kabukoba & Young (1992) bear repeating: 35% of midwives were not wearing gloves during vaginal deliveries. Midwives who say that they have never had anyone infected with HIV in their unit are probably deceiving themselves. It is merely that they have not known the women were infected. It is only by applying universal precautions that midwives will be able to protect themselves. Such practice has other benefits too. It would reduce the sense being treated differently, which can have a very isolating effect on those who are infected.

## Innovations in labour

Some of the recent innovations in labour, such as water births, raise additional dilemmas for the midwife in the management of labour. The guidelines state categorically that staff should wear sensible protective clothing for delivery, to prevent contact with body fluids such as blood and liquor. Some of the water baths or birthing pools in use make this rather difficult. The present trend to encourage women to have control and choice during their childbirth experience is contradicted if there is an arbitrary decision to exclude certain categories of women from such amenities as a birthing pool.

## POSTPARTUM CARE

At this stage in the expansion of the pandemic, just over a decade since the recognition of the disease, the most rapidly growing group of infected individuals is women of childbearing age. Thus the care given by midwives to women who are infected and to their infants, who may be so, is of vital importance. One estimate of the mother–infant transmission rate is 30% (Valente & Main 1990). This estimate, however, is hampered by the difficulties of diagnosing the infected infant. As already mentioned, babies may be born with maternal antibodies and as a consequence, HIV tests (which are of antibodies) will return positive results during the first 15–18 months. Subsequently, the children may be seronegative on testing, indicating that they have not been infected.

## Breast feeding

The change of the infant's serological status, from positive to negative, has implications for the decision whether to breast feed or not. As the presence of the virus has been demonstrated in breast milk, there is a possibility that breast feeding may infect the infant that has not been infected by any other route. This has to be considered when advising women about the method of feeding their babies.

The latest information and advice from WHO suggests that where infants are at greater risk of death from gastrointestinal conditions than if they become HIV-infected, then breast feeding should be encouraged (Finger 1992). Such conditions are more common in developing countries. Where the risk of death from gastroenteritis is less than the risk of HIV, then breast feeding should be discouraged. Quite apart from the worries about illness and death in what is normally a happy occasion, midwives who spend most of their time encouraging breast feeding, can now be in the unhappy position of having to advise against it.

## Postpartum infections

A number of reports suggest that there is an increase in the incidence of postpartum infection and illness among all women and especially those with HIV. There is also a tendency for perineal and abdominal wounds to heal poorly (Gloeb et al 1988). Postpartum haemorrhage may occur more frequently among women who are taking AZT because it has the side effect of thrombocytopenia.

## Precautions for midwives during postpartum care

As with the intrapartum period, the risk of infection is considerable postnatally. In hospital it is essential that there are clear policies for the disposal of all items involving body fluids and that these policies are firmly enforced. It has always been part of the midwive's role to teach mothers to care for themselves. If the policies are applied universally, there is no need to emphasise that the precautions are taken in relation to HIV.

The careful management of blood spillage should be incorporated into all postnatal care as HIV is not the only blood-borne virus. Women with HIV may also have sexually transmitted diseases, and the risk of hepatitis B is a major concern in the care of women who are drug abusers.

Ordinary household bleach will kill viruses effectively and its use should be encouraged as part of the domestic routine. The proper disposal of perineal pads should be taught in hospital and also be encouraged in the home. This is not only necessary to protect the family but also for refuse workers who have to dispose of domestic rubbish.

## CARE OF WOMEN WITH KNOWN HIV INFECTION

### Counselling and advice

In addition to the preventative measures for all women, those who are known to carry the HIV will require further counselling and advice. Midwives need to be able to advise about the symptoms of HIV progression as the early recognition of the latter holds the best hope of successful management of opportunistic infections. Symptoms such as loss of weight, persistent sore throat, unusual vaginal discharge or cough are significant.

Advice on contraception and safer sex will be important, not only to prevent a further pregnancy which would have enormous physical and emotional consequences for the family, but also to minimise the risk of the more aggressive forms of vaginal infection such as candida. Such infections are often difficult to eradicate in these circumstances.

#### Contraception advice

Unfortunately there are advantages and disadvantages to all common methods of contraception. For example, the cap, sponge and intrauterine device are all foreign bodies which are a potential risk for creating a portal of entry for the HIV. A combination of methods needs to be used, to provide maximum contraception with a maximum barrier effect.

The midwife giving advice must not omit the safer sex aspect.

The sexual practices which carry a risk of transmitting the HIV infection are all those which involve exchange of body fluids. To reduce the risk, some of these behaviours need to be modified. It is not possible to ensure that preventative measures will be used satisfactorily if either of the partners is under the influence of alcohol or drugs.

### Advice on prevention of other infections

Apart from sexually acquired infections, the HIV-positive woman must be advised on all aspects of prevention of other infections, for herself and other members of her family who may also be infected. This includes the new baby, although midwives' advice should be the same for all women. Women have to be taught the sources of infection, such as those transmitted by food (e.g. chickens and salmonella), domestic animals (e.g. cats and toxoplasmosis) or shared toilet articles (e.g. razors).

### Health education

In addition to teaching women to avoid infection, it is important to teach the HIV-positive woman how to take active steps to keep well. This includes a sound plan for the nutrition of the family and a lifestyle which incorporates suitable exercise and relaxation. Advice to give up smoking may be excellent and would be a major step in the fight against infection, but for those who are facing death within the foreseeable future, it may be very difficult. Such advice is given to women antenatally, but it is also appropriate postnatally because it will apply for the rest of their lives.

## Subsequent monitoring of HIV infection

Women will need to be followed up with frequent gynaecological examinations, as the disease frequently follows a gynaecological route. After the postnatal visit at 6 weeks there should be regular cervical smears, because the rate of abnormal cervical cytology is increased in HIV-positive women and the progress of malignant cervical conditions is much accelerated. Some American centres recommend smears every 4–6 months (Allen 1990). Women who have a continuing drug abuse problem will require special care to maintain their health as far as is possible.

## CARE OF THE INFANT

At present the statistics from the USA are the most useful for countries like the UK. These indicate that most cases of HIV infection in children were acquired perinatally, and that if the current trend continues, AIDS and HIV infection will become one of the top five causes of death in children under 5 years in the USA.

The infection follows three pathways: across the placenta; from exposure to maternal body fluid at delivery; and postnatally via maternal body fluid including breast milk. It has not been demonstrated that delivering by caesarean section alters the risk of infection (Viscarello 1990)

Because the passively acquired maternal antibodies may be present at birth and for up to 18 months afterwards, it is difficult to confirm that the infant is infected. Babies may remain well for several years after birth but many develop symptoms of AIDS in the first 2 years. The median age at which the first signs of the disease appear is 9 months.

The signs of HIV infection in children include failure to thrive, lymphadenopathy hepatosplenomegaly, oral candida, and developmental problems affecting the central nervous system. More severe symptoms include meningitis and pneumocystis carinii pneumonia. Infants whose development as a fetus has been impaired by maternal viraemia follow a much more rapid course of the HIV disease.

The women will need to be advised that signs such as increased irritability, poor feeding, failure to thrive, cough and oral thrush should be reported so that the best care can be given as early as possible. The general management of infants of known seropositive women should include increased paediatric follow-up. All infants should be treated as seronegative until proved otherwise and every possible precaution should be taken to reduce the risk of infecting a non-infected infant.

## RUMOURS AND DIVERSIONS

During the progress of this disease, into all levels of society and all countries of the world, there have been many short-lived diversions. These have been mainly in the area of cures. The amount of research work being carried out on AIDS worldwide is considerable, and is often in competition with research on the more common causes of mortality for scarce funds. There may be hope of a cure to be found in herbal remedies, with the search ranging from the common British daisy to exotic inhabitants of the rain forest.

The Eighth International Conference on AIDS in Amsterdam in July 1992 were told of a dramatic discovery of a case of CD4 deficiency without evidence of HIV infection. Other cases were then brought forward and discussed. The media reports created public reaction, claims of a cover-up and concerns for public safety. The causative factor in these new cases was not identified; some suggested a new virus, others proposed this to be a new facet of the HIV. However, we have known other causes of immune deficiency for a long time. The research work continues.

Professor Peter Duesberg of the University of California has challenged the hypothesis that HIV causes AIDS and an ongoing debate is in progress between the majority of AIDS experts and this minority view (Duesberg 1987).

The knowledge base about this infection, and the different manifestation of the disease we call AIDS, is limited at present. Midwives should be alert to all aspects of the pandemic in order to contribute positively to the body of knowledge as we move forward to combat the problems this condition presents and will continue to present for the foreseeable future.

## LOOKING TO THE FUTURE

Where will the AIDS crisis place midwives in the future? Will there be a public demand for segregation? If so, which group, infected or non-infected, should be segregated? Will the difficulties of identification remain, so that it will be impossible to make the distinction between one group and the other?

If midwives are to manage all women in the same way then new guidelines must be developed, because some women are already infected and more will become so. As their babies may not be infected, it will be vital to prevent such infection. These considerations require a review of some of the common practices in the delivery suite, especially those which create a portal between the baby and the mother's body fluids. Procedures such as the application of scalp electrodes, fetal blood sampling and ventouse extraction need to be examined rigorously, using the criterion of the overall welfare of the baby. Such a review should extend to procedures performed immediately after delivery and before the baby is bathed such as injections and heel stabs. Should the bathing of the baby be carried out immediately after the birth? The care of the umbilical cord is another issue requiring review.

The procedures midwives undertake must be safe for every single baby. It is not possible to know at the onset of labour which mothers are positive, which are in the biological time gap and which are negative. Granted this fact, if its implications are heeded, then logically the only safe practice in labour is to ban the use of scalp electrodes. Is there any maternity unit that has changed its policy to follow this logic? Is there any maternity unit where this is even being considered? How do the staff who have to make such policies balance this proposal with the increasing incidence of litigation? If the public equate good care with machines, will policies designed to prevent a small number of babies from becoming infected with HIV, be regarded as negligence?

A further facet of this ambivalence is the present enthusiasm for water births. Despite some adverse publicity at the end of 1993 in the UK, the question was about the well-being of the baby at birth rather than concern about an increased risk of HIV transmission. In the present climate of offering choice to women is this a choice that should be offered? If choice is to be an informed choice, not only is there need for public education but also there is a need to confirm whether water births do, in fact, carry an increased risk of infection.

One consultant obstetrician has described midwifery as a 'blood sport'. While I find this remark lacking in taste it does graphically portray the difficulties midwives can encounter in trying to contain body fluids during labour and delivery.

I believe midwives in UK are suffering from a peculiar form of apathy. There is a danger that it is more comfortable to mentally confine this disease only to the gay men in whom it was first recognised. At the beginning of the 1990s well known people are developing AIDS and their deaths are making headline news. The length of time between infection and AIDS is variable, as the mean is 5.5 years and maximum recorded to date is 14 years. Consequently those whose deaths are news today are still mainly gay men. This is to be expected because they were members of the first group to be infected. But there lies the hazard. In the public consciousness HIV/AIDS is still a 'gay disease'. It is only when it affects the man or the woman or the baby next door that the public at large, including midwives, will begin to realise the personal impact.

Towards the end of 1990 a consultant in genitourinary medicine lectured to a group of student midwives from a town in the north-west of England on the subject of HIV infection. The north-west is second only to London in the frequency of this condition. He asked them how long they thought it was going to be before the first HIV-positive woman came for antenatal care in the unit in which they worked. On receipt of a variety of predictions, he informed them such a woman had already delivered in their unit. Had they known? Of course not. It was only because the woman was also a genitourinary patient that he knew; otherwise her condition would have been completely unknown. She was not the only one in that unit nor in any of the maternity units throughout the UK.

This same consultant further upset the applecart by telling the student midwives that the local 'gay' clubs were much frequented by married men. They did not even know that the town had a gay club and began to wonder about the weekly 'night out with the boys' common among their married menfolk.

This anecdote may have its funny aspects but the issues are serious. The situation facing midwives is not unique within health care but there are aspects which make it especially significant. The population midwives care for are young and, by definition, sexually active; they are bound to be more at risk than their grandmothers, (but we must not discount grandmothers either) even if they do not come into one of the well known risk groups. The process of birth abounds in body fluids and HIV can be present in most of them.

Midwives now have to confront a range of issues not considered important 10 years ago. Is the splash of blood on the floor of the delivery room or the sluice, a risk to the staff? How long does the virus live in dried blood spots? If, as seems probable, the answer is 3–4 hours, what does this mean for midwives, cleaners, and porters? Will gloves protect the staff from blood penetration as they clear it up? Gloves do not always provide protection, so are the hands in the them always free from breaks in the skin? If there are skin cracks or breaks, are staff concerned enough, aware enough, to cover them before putting on gloves? It may seem to be turning the clock back to suggest that hands should be inspected as staff come on duty as they used to be 30 years ago, but maybe it is necessary.

Midwives must now care for themselves and for their colleagues in a way that was not necessary previously. When faced with a fatal infection it is essential to behave in a way that reflects the reality. Although discussion with colleagues demonstrates that they are not ignorant of these matters they truly do seem to be protected by an 'it won't happen to me' attitude, an attitude that could lead to a complacency that is fatal. There have already been midwives and obstetricians who have died of AIDS. Although the publicity surrounding these deaths has not been in the public interest, it might at least increase awareness among those in the maternity services that this is not an issue for gay men only.

How long can midwives in the UK go on like this? We need to waken from our apathy and make sure it does not happen to us because 'our public needs us' and may need us to return our practice more and more to the community setting as the demand for acute high-tech beds for AIDS patients increases.

## CONCLUSION

While discovery of a cure is always possible, the development of a cure or even a vaccine is some distance away, and in the intervening time there will be increasing numbers of infected individuals. It may be that our best hope lies in genetic engineering. An experienced worker in this field, Professor Mann of the Harvard School of Public Health, regards the pandemic as a global health crisis and postulates that this crisis should become a central defining principle in guiding national and global purpose towards the WHO ideal that 'health is one of the fundamental rights of every human being' and that 'the health of all peoples is fundamental to the attainment of peace'. Not only do midwives subscribe to this ideal, they are also in a position to contribute to it.

REFERENCES

Ades A E, Parker S, Berry T, Holland F J, Davison C F, Cubitt D, Hjelm M, Wilcox A H, Hudson C N, Briggs M, Tedder R S, Peckham C S 1991 Prevalence of

Maternal HIV-1 in Thames region: results from anonymous unlinked neonatal testing. Lancet ii: 1562–1564

Allen M 1990, Inpatient maternity care of women infected with HIV. Obstetric and Gynecology Clinics of North America 17: 557–570

Bastin N, Tamayo O W, Tinkle M B, Amaya M A, Trejo L R, Herrera C 1992 HIV disease and pregnancy. Part 3: post partum care of the HIV positive woman and her newborn. Journal of Obstetric Gynecologic and Neonatal Nursing 21(2): 105–111

Department of Health 1991 Recommendations of the Expert Advisory Group on AIDS. HMSO, London

Duesberg P H 1987 Retroviruses as carinogens and pathogens: expectations and reality. Cancer Research 47: 1199–1220 Cited in: Stewart G 1993 Predictable and preventable? Nursing Times 89(26): 29–32, 30 June – 6 July

Efantis J, Sinclair B P 1990, Inpatient maternity care for HIV infection in women and the newborn. In: Sinclair B P, McCormick A (eds) NAACOG Clinical issues in perinatal and women's health nursing. Antepartum Management of Pregnant Women with HIV Infection 1: 47–52

Eighth International Conference on AIDS 1992 Lancet 340, 1 August 1992

English National Board for Nursing, Midwifery and Health Visiting 1987 In: Marson S (ed) AIDS: meeting the challenge. ENB, London

Finger W R 1992, Should the threat of HIV affect breastfeeding? Network 13(2): 12–14

Gloeb D J, O'Sullivan J O, Efantis J 1988 HIV infection in women: the effects of HIV in pregnancy. American Journal of Obstetrics and Gynecology 159: 756–761

Kabukoba J, Young P 1992 Midwifery and body fluid contamination. British Medical Journal 305: 226

Koonin L M, Ellerbrock T V, Atrash H K, Rogers M F, Smith J C, Hogue C J, Harris M A, Chavkn W, Parker A L, Halpin G J 1989 Pregnancy associated deaths due to AIDS in the United States. Journal of the American Medical Association 261: 1306–1309

Mann J 1992 AIDS in the 1990s. Journal of the Royal Society of Health 112(3): 143–148

Nanda D 1990 HIV infection in women in the USA. Obstetrics and Gynecology Clinics of North America 17: 617–625

Public Health Laboratory Service 1992 News Release 24.8.1992: Monthly AIDS figures, CDSC, London

Public Health Laboratory Service 1994 Communitable Diseases Report, CDSC London 4(7): 34

Scattergood S 1992 A survey of midwives' use of eye protection in delivery rooms. Unpublished

Tierney A J, Bond S, Rhodes T, Philips P 1990 HIV infection, AIDS and community nursing staff in Scotland. Health Bulletin 48(3): 114–123

Tinkle M B Amaya M A Tamayo O W 1992 HIV disease and pregnancy. Part 1: epidemiology, parthogenesis and natural history. Journal of Obstetric, Gynecologic, and Neonatal Nursing 21(2): 86–93

Valente P, Main E 1990 Role of the placenta in perinatal transmission of HIV. Obstetrics and Gynecology Clinics of North America 17: 607–615

Viscarello R 1990 AIDS Natural history and prognosis Obstetrics and Gynecology Clinics of North America 17: 545–555

World Health Organisation Regional Office for Europe 1992 AIDS in Europe: the challenge for today and tomorrow. Summary report. Journal of Advanced Nursing 17: 888–891

Yarchoan R, Mitsuya H, Broder S 1989, Clinical and basic advances in the antiretroviral therapy of HIV infection. American Journal of Medicine 87: 191–200

## FURTHER READING

Acosta Y M, Goodwin C, Amaya M A, Tinkle M B, Acosta E, Jaquez I 1992 HIV disease and pregnancy. Part 2: antepartum and intrapartum care. Journal of Obstetric, Gynecologic, and Neonatal Nursing 21(2): 97–103
Kay K 1989 AIDS: a global concern Midwifery. 5: 84–95

# 13

# Midwives, nurses and doctors: interprofessional relationships

*Sharon Cochrane*

## INTRODUCTION

At the outset of this project the literature search for this chapter revealed some interesting factors. There was a bewildering array of references on the subject of nurse–doctor collaborative practice and interprofessional relationships. There were no articles or research papers on the relationship between nurses and midwives. There were none on the relationship between midwives and doctors. This was baffling and posed the question: 'Is this because nothing has been written on the subject?' Or, is it perhaps the result of the supposition that midwifery is merely a branch of nursing?

The relationship between midwives and doctors has for centuries been an uneasy one. Despite being complementary professions involved in the process of childbirth they are often projected as antagonists in the control of childbirth and of the childbearing women they serve.

The problems are universal, complex and have their origins far back in history. The relative positions of the two professions within society are now culturally enshrined; challenges to the status quo have done little to establish midwives as independent practitioners on a par with doctors.

## AN HISTORICAL PERSPECTIVE

### Midwifery in early societies

In attempting to discover the origins of medicine, midwifery and obstetrics it is necessary to look back at the origins of humanity. From the Paleolithic Age, men and women formed pair bonds, and it is believed that men assisted women in childbirth at this time. In the Neolithic Age, humankind began to organise small communal hunting groups, and women assisted each other in childbirth. Towards the end of the Ice Age, when the climate improved, larger family groups began to settle leading to an agricultural and primitive farming lifestyle, and away from nomadic hunter-gathering. With increasing social organisation, women replaced men as childbirth attendants (Towler & Bramall 1986).

Primitive humanity with its dependence on nature, feared and worshipped elemental forces. The mysterious processes of child-birth and fertility were attributed to the magical powers of the gods. Normal deliveries proceeded under the guidance of elderly experienced women, but in difficult labours primitive shamans were called upon to invoke the assistance of the gods. Labour was considered a voluntary act, and the shaman would attempt to coax or frighten the child from the birth canal into the outside world. Elaborate and grisly rituals to expedite delivery are well chronicled. Throughout the world, women, when giving birth to their children whether helped at all, by men or by women, depended upon the degree of social development of the community (Roush 1979).

From very early times, it becomes evident that the religious bodies of all cultures took an active role in governing medical and midwifery practice. Women as traditional birth attendants, were already dealing only with uncomplicated labours, and assistance was sought from priests, rabbis, Hindu Brahmans and doctors whenever difficulties arose. Women in all these cultures deferred to men as the 'educated' leaders of the community. These traditions continue in the midwife's Code of Practice, in the detection of abnormal conditions in mother and child and the procurement of medical assistance, and are considered the basis of good contemporary practice.

### Written history

For primitive man, with language also came literacy. Many cultures forbade women to learn reading skills which in turn prevented them from writing. Much written work of men survives to enhance literate history, whilst the unwritten body of women's knowledge has been lost or merely ascribed the status of folklore.

Writings concerning midwifery and childbirth can be traced back as far as 4000 BC in the Tao Te Ching, and 2200 in the Kahun papyrus.

The next most famous reference to midwives occurred around 1500 BC in the Biblical passage from the book of Exodus, Chapter 1. Against the decree of the King of Egypt, the midwives to the Hebrews had allowed male infants to survive after birth. The King, who feared an uprising from the enslaved Hebrews, had ordered male infanticide at birth. The King called the midwives to give account of their actions. They said: 'Hebrew women are not like Egyptian women; for they are vigorous, and they give birth before the midwife can get to them'. As a reward for their endeavours, verses 20 and 21 state: 'God was good to the midwives . . . and established households for them'.

In 1400 BC Hindu writings described in detail every possible action to be taken if the midwife were presented with anything other than a cephalic presentation, and had to seek the aid of a doctor.

## From the Greeks and Romans to the Dark Ages

In Greece in 1400 BC midwives were menopausal mothers themselves and there were two grades of midwife. The first was a birth attendant and matchmaker, the second was a senior midwife of doctor status. Plato in his writings mentions Phaenarete, probably less well known for her proficiency as a midwife than as the mother of Socrates.

Greek medical influences were adopted by the Romans, and Rome imported midwives from the Greek and Alexandrian schools. Hierophilus famous for his description of the ovary, wrote a book on midwifery around 300 BC. Rome's contributions to gynaecological and obstetric writing and practice came in 98 AD through the Ephesian, Soranus, who emerged as one of the first specialists in the field. Galen, from 130 AD, further advanced medicine but wrote little on obstetrics, so Soranus continued to be the major influence for the next 1500 years. Ambroise Paré reintroduced podalic version to obstetric practice, as first described by Soranus, 1400 years earlier.

From the decline of the Greek and Roman empires through the Dark and Middle Ages, few advances in obstetrics and gynaecology were made. Midwives did what was necessary and called for help when the birth process failed to proceed. The ancient world was constantly at war, and only a few medical documents survived the sacking of the great Alexandrian library when the Saracens conquered Egypt around 640 AD. With the rise of Islam came another period of suspended animation of obstetric and gynaecological knowledge. Religious law forbade the examination of women by men.

## The Middle Ages and the Renaissance

Medicine again began to advance after 800 AD. Charlemagne instigated the setting up of schools through the monasteries and cathedrals, and medicine was again recognised as a subject worthy of study.

The first medieval medical school was set up in Salerno in the 11th century, and it was there in the 12th century that anatomy was again studied. The emergence of the universities in the 12th and 13th centuries developed law, medicine, art and theology as separate disciplines. Women were not admitted to the universities to study.

Originally the Church was the controlling body. The university teachers, aware of the restricting power of the church, came into conflict with the bishops. The problem was resolved when the bishops granted licences to teach, and the scholars had control of who entered their particular guild.

There then came two degrees of licenciate and master. The teachers of theology and medicine were both referred to as doctors. The modern concept of the medical doctor did not emerge until several centuries later.

Through Church and State, formal learning remained a male preserve. The restriction of medical practice to those from university faculties began to appear. Statutes and a papal bull were promulgated by 1421 in England, and medical practice was limited to medical school graduates.

The rise of medicine saw the decline of the status and practice of midwifery. The midwife, in common with her clients, was mainly illiterate and of low social status. The stigma of the profession at that time did not encourage the involvement of learned men, and midwives actively guarded against men in the delivery chamber. This separation lead to a gulf between the professions.

The Church insisted on the baptism of all infants dead or alive, and the government began to take an interest in the welfare of the populace. In Paris in 1560 the first statute of midwifery was passed. Training, licensing and registration were administered by a doctor, two representatives of the King and two approved midwives of high status. Following apprenticeship and cross-examination by the panel above, a successful candidate was given permission to practise midwifery in the community. She was allowed to advertise her services by fixing a plaque of her profession on her door.

It is almost inconceivable that this statute was passed during the most sinister age of witchhunting throughout Europe. Back in England, midwives found themselves in an unenviable position where their activities were prohibited by law because they were unlicensed practitioners 'of medicine and other useful skills' (Towler & Bramall 1986). A normal delivery classified the midwife as a 'white witch', and the delivery of a stillborn or deformed infant, or a maternal death could condemn the midwife to a gruesome death.

## From the 16th to the 19th century

A social conscience gradually awoke in the 16th century, and was marked in England by the passing of the first Poor Law in 1601. Midwives were licensed through the church, and had to be wise and discreet, have expertise and be worthy to hold the office of midwife.

The civil war had led to a re-emergence of the Church of England and Episcopal licensing, though still practised, was giving way to municipal licensing. Licences were expensive. In 1662 the price was 82½ pence, and by 1714 it had risen to 8 pounds and 40 pence. For the majority of midwives these sums of money were beyond their reach and so many remained unlicensed. In the middle of the 17th century men re-entered the childbirth arena. The first of note was William Harvey who wrote an English textbook on midwifery in 1651. Through his studies, obstetrics was given a scientific basis. Following Harvey, Percival Willoughby wrote a comprehensive description of the state of midwifery. He saw education of midwives as crucial to effect better outcomes to pregnancy and childbirth. He stated: 'A woman is not born a midwife, it is education with practice that teaches her experience' (Towler & Bramall 1986). He observed women of the working classes and concluded that labour often proceeded without the necessity for any intervention.

The next major development came from the Chamberlen family who introduced forceps to midwifery practice. These men were licensed through the Company of Barber Surgeons, having been refused entry to the Company of Physicians as they did not have an Oxford or Cambridge university education. Divisions in the midwifery profession arose as some male midwives adopted the indiscriminate use of forceps. Few female midwives were well educated at the time; the majority were perceived to be ignorant peasants practising in rural communities.

In 1671 the first textbook written by an English midwife was published (Donnison 1988). The book was entitled *The Midwives Book* and was written by Jane Sharp, 'Practitioner of the Art of Midwifery above thirty years'. She was aware that although male midwives were often only brought in to difficult labours, their assumedly greater education, and the preference for their practice by the upper classes, meant that they had the potential to usurp the female midwives from their traditional role. They also sought much larger financial returns for their services.

William Smellie was an eminent practitioner of midwifery who advocated the education of women separately from men. He felt that allowances should be made for women as the weaker sex. Despite his condescending attitude, he did recognise the necessity of obstetricians and midwives working much more closely together.

Gradually more books about midwifery were written by men and women and the two professions developed separately.

Doctors established lying-in hospitals in the 19th century. The Colleges of Physicians and Surgeons called for regulations to govern untrained medical practitioners, including male midwives. 1813 saw attempts to pass a Bill through Parliament to regulate female midwives' practice. In 1815 the Society of Apothecaries persuaded the College of Surgeons to restrict the practice of midwifery by men to holders of their diploma.

They did very well until the stillbirth and maternal death of Princess Charlotte. She was attended by an obstetrician and two physicians; the assumption that female midwives were incompetent and doctors competent, lost some of its momentum.

## The 20th century

The first Midwives' Act of 1902, in England, set up the Central Midwives' Board to provide better training and regulate practice. The work to politicise midwifery had been carried out by the Midwives' Institute and had taken 22 years to be reflected in the law of the United Kingdom.

As midwifery began to establish itself in law and by recognised training in the UK persecution continued in the USA. Under intense pressure from the medical profession, state after state in America passed laws outlawing midwifery and restricting the practice of obstetrics to doctors (Inch 1989). There is renewed interest in midwifery today, in the USA and Canada, and new training programmes are being devised, with midwifery qualifications being recognised in some states.

In the UK, 90 years on from the original Midwives' Act of 1902, the Midwives' Legislation Group is once more seeking a separate Parliamentary Bill, leading to a new Act of Parliament, to recognise the unique role of midwifery and the midwife, separate from both obstetrics and nursing. History does repeat itself.

## NURSES AND MIDWIVES

The interprofessional relationships between nurses and midwives are quite interesting, and there are antagonisms between the respective Colleges.

Nurses tend to perceive midwives as condescending in their attitudes, and that midwives consider themselves superior. This may have originated from the time when most nurses went on to do midwifery training after nursing, regardless of whether they intended to practise. This also helped to give midwifery the appearance of being a branch of the nursing profession. Many 'sister' grade posts required prospective candidates to have the dual qualification. As more specific nursing courses have became available, fewer nurses have undertaken midwifery training purely to obtain the certificate at the end of the course. It was ludicrous for oncology or renal specialists to be qualified in a profession they had no interest in.

Midwives' perceptions of nurses are that they are subservient to doctors. They believe that nurses are doubly conditioned to play the subservient role: first by society in general, and secondly by the medical establishment (Pizurki et al 1987). Nurses are seen, as a profession, to envy the practitioner status midwives have held for some time and to have attempted to establish themselves on a par with midwives; through accountability, and by attaining prescribing rights they are attempting to emulate midwives.

Both sets of perceptions are inaccurate, and merely serve to fuel hostilities and divide two prestigious professions that should be natural allies. Accountability cannot be delegated in either profession. The ratio of nurses to midwives in the UK is approximately 5:1; the two groups are not superior or inferior to each other, they are just different. In order to value the unique qualities of each profession, there needs to be an open dialogue in which it can be established that equality does not demand that they are the same, and that diversity is valid.

The same processes can be applied to the nurse–midwife, midwife–doctor and doctor–nurse attitudes. Trying to understand how we can contribute to care, and why we work in the way we do will be an important preliminary in re-establishing the relationship (Malby 1989). Two-way educational processes are crucial to avoid future deadlocks and the continuation of professional rivalries.

## MIDWIVES AND DOCTORS

In the UK today, midwifery is a predominantly female profession and the medical profession is still predominantly male, although there are some male midwives and female obstetricians.

The issue is not simply a clash of feminism versus paternalism, as neither feminist nor paternalistic attitudes are confined rigidly to women or men respectively. The nurturing nature of men is often underestimated and only comes to the fore in an environment in which the individual man is valued and nurtured, and where empathy is developed and encouraged. The paternalistic capacity of women thrives in an environment where emotion, nature and nurture are viewed with less regard than the application of logic, science and medicalisation. The mantle of male values and attitudes develops as a survival technique where the old adage 'if you can't beat them, join them' rings most true.

Popular and media culture has frequent reference to romantic attachments between women and their gynaecologists. Doctors are often portrayed as young and handsome or elderly and kindly, occasionally frosty. Nurses on the other hand are stereotyped into the 'sex-kitten' or 'old battle-axe' moulds; there are very few references to male nurses. Midwives tend to be imagined as middle-aged and buxom, with white, curly permed hair. They either ride old fashioned sturdy black bicycles or drive elderly blue mini cars and carry ubiquitous 'Gladstone' bags. Each inaccurate image reinforces existing attitudes in the minds of the public and issues subliminal endorsements of gender stereotyping. It may appear flippant to use such illustrations but they do affect the mode and manner of relationships between health care workers and their clients, and the interprofessional relationships that doctors, nurses and midwives have with each other.

Obstetrics and gynaecology are virtually inseparable today with a very high profile in Europe, the United States, Canada and Australia. In Britain, doctors undertake the joint role of obstetrician and gynaecologist, moving between the two disciplines as if they were one. It would seem errant to combine physiology and pathology, in two separate situations, with the only common denominator being the gender of the patient. Perhaps the free movement of operators goes some way to explaining the medical models applied to parturition.

Gynaecology is perceived as dynamic and innovative in terms of surgical technique, and largely devoid of the inconvenience and potentially litigious aspects associated with obstetric practice. Paternalism in gynaecology is the root from which misogyny in obstetrics originates. The medicalisation of midwives occurs when the same values of pathology are accepted, and applied to midwifery. The hospital hierarchy maintains the doctor in a superior position to the midwife who, by an elaborate system of policies and procedures and the Midwives' Rules and Code of Conduct, remains subordinate.

## THE CONTEMPORARY SETTING IN THE UNITED KINGDOM

### Where midwives work

The current situation in the UK is that the vast majority of midwives are employed by local health authorities within a hospital setting, and a smaller number are employed in the same system to work in the community. There are a number of midwives employed in the rapidly expanding private sector. An even smaller number of midwives work independently of the National Health Service (NHS) and private sector systems, undertaking total care in partnership with women and their families and providing a home birth service.

From figures obtained from the United Kingdom Central Council for Nursing, Midwifery and Health Visiting (UKCC), in 1991 there were:

104 423 midwives on the register, including 77 male midwives
 34 626 midwives practising, including 36 male midwives
     46 self-employed (independent) midwives of whom
           44 were in England
            1 was in Wales
            1 was in Northern Ireland
   204 GP practice nurses who had notified their intention to practise as midwives
   814 registered midwife teachers

Unfortunately there was no breakdown available as to the exact number of midwives employed in the private and public sectors.

### Hospital and home births

The development of the NHS after the second World War brought the services of the general practitioner (GP), obstetrician and midwife within the reach of all pregnant women, regardless of social class. The trend towards the provision of a hospital bed as a right for every woman began following the Peel Report in 1970 which advocated 100% hospital births 'for the safety of the mother and baby' (Peel Committee Report 1970). The government of the day implemented the report, the beds justified their existence by constant usage and, by 1972, 92% of births in the UK occurred in hospital.

Home confinement began to be viewed as the unwise choice of the ill-informed. Many women requesting a home birth still find a less than enthusiastic reception from their family GP. In fact, for some, the response is quite hostile despite the recommendations of the House of Commons Health Committee Report on Maternity Services (Select Committee on Health 1992):

We recommend that the Department of Health take steps to impress upon all GPs their duty to facilitate the wishes of women, especially in respect of their choice of place of birth and their right to midwifery-only care. Family Services Health Authorities (FSHA) should also take steps to impress upon all GP practices that it is wrong to remove a woman from their list solely because they wish to have a home confinement, or midwifery-only care, and we recommend appropriate safeguards to prevent this.

We recommend that it be a duty placed upon all GP practices to have in place arrangements for women to have a home confinement with GP cover or midwife-only cover if they so desire.

## Confusion between nursing and midwifery

Nursing and midwifery are separate but complementary professions, in a similar way to medicine and dentistry. There is often confusion amongst both the medical profession and the general public as to the roles of the two professions. Many midwives have experience of being referred to as 'nurse' by their colleagues and their clients. In Scotland and Ireland this is the norm and rarely challenged, and in the USA 'nurse-midwife' is the legal registration title of midwives.

Perhaps some of the confusion can be explained by the fact that many midwives have entered the profession by first becoming nurses, and that in most generic nurse training there is a maternity component. Perhaps the similarity of style of uniform, job title (staff nurse/staff midwife, sister/charge nurse) and the association of hospital with a 'sick' model have all contributed to the general lack of understanding. In some parts of this country the job of district nurse/midwife involves one person, and in extremely outlying rural communities one person may undertake the triple role of district nurse/midwife/health visitor (for a single salary).

## Professional autonomy of nurses and midwives and 'doctors' orders'

The phenomenon of 'doctors' orders' can also lead to problems. An 'order' in the army is used by an officer to march foot soldiers into the path live ammunition (Manthey 1989). In the United States, according to Manthey, 'the courts require nurses to obey doctors' orders when they are correct. Failure to discriminate between correct and incorrect orders places the nurse at risk of being sued for malpractice or negligence'.

Both nurses and midwives may be in the difficult situation of not sharing the same professional opinion as their medical colleagues over the appropriate choice of treatment or mode of action in a given situation. Physicians and nurses place different values on specific aspects of the health care continuum (Morgan & McCann 1983). It is difficult for a nurse or midwife to be assertive in the interests of the patient or client without incurring the disapproval of the doctor. The questioning of the doctor is sometimes interpreted with suspicion, and occasionally as an insult to the rank and position of the doctor in the medical hierarchy.

There are provisions within the nurses' and midwives' Codes of Practice for the nurse or midwife to refuse to be involved in any situation which they may consider not to be in the best interests of the patient or client. However, there are few situations in which all the issues are clear, and professionals can find themselves with doubts rather than convictions, and compliance an easier bedfellow than confrontation. The gradual erosion of confidence from repeated exposure to situations of this kind can lead the nurse or midwife to practice in a non-confrontational manner, reinforcing a subordinate role.

It is interesting to note that whilst applauding the virtues of free-thinking individuals within the health service, many managers prefer employees to share their own concepts and ideals. The nurse or midwife who comes into conflict may find him/herself alone, an anachronism within a system which perpetuates itself in all its imperfections.

There are changes within the professions, and gradually some midwives are beginning to challenge the old order and work more autonomously, in partnership with their clients, within the existing structure of the Health Service.

## The consumers' voice

In spite of the gradual increase in midwives' autonomy mentioned above, it is sad but true that most of the changes in attitude toward parturient women have come through their own expression of dissatisfaction with highly technological and impersonal services provided by health care professionals. Routine procedures such as electronic fetal heart monitoring, amniotomy, induction of labour, episiotomy, enemas and pubic shaves were certainly not popular with the women who endured them.

The women themselves formed pressure groups such as the National Childbirth Trust and the Association for the Improvement of Maternity Services in the 1970s, and it was through them that their collective voices were heard by professionals and government alike.

For decades the woman's right to choice has not been perceived as valid by either midwives or obstetricians and 'safety' has been cited as the main objection to the introduction of more liberal practices. Professionals have felt seriously threatened by the often vocal and assertive client. Now that consumer groups have ready access to research findings and are more critically astute than previously, researchers can find themselves called to account by both their clients and their peers.

## Research by nurses and midwives

Nurses and midwives have also found the need to examine their practices, and research projects have multiplied in the last 10 years.

A significant number of midwife/nurse researchers have opted for a medical model of research for the reason that, in order to be taken seriously by the medical establishment, projects must be presented in the style of those undertaken by doctors. However, many aspects of midwifery care lend themselves more readily to qualitative, rather than quantitative, examination.

### Language issues

Power comes from the ability to express oneself articulately and assertively. Those in the medical profession are, by and large, more articulate. Generally medical education is of a higher standard and encourages one to be forceful and analytical (Smith 1987). A good example of the differences in education is that medical students are taught about haemaglobinopathies and nursing and midwifery students learn about anaemias. Simple enough one might think, but this kind of approach means that the nurse/midwife then has to learn a completely new language in order to access medical information.

The situation is compounded when nurses and midwives emulate doctors when writing research theses themselves. The language becomes self-limiting, verbose and, at times, completely unintelligible. The substance of the thesis is lost to the reader as the writer attempts to impress.

Words can be extremely powerful tools. The language we use gives subtle clues to our attitudes and the ideologies that underline midwifery care (Leap 1992). For instance, there has been a lot of discussion about autonomous practice and midwives giving 'autonomy' to women. It is not possible to give a woman autonomy, it is intrinsic; it is possible to take it away. For midwives to talk of 'allowing' women to deliver their babies in their preferred environment or position constitutes an oppression of the weaker by the weak, just as when doctors 'allow' midwives not to perform amniotomy in early labour on 'their' patients.

If we are truly dedicated to research-based practice, and if we are really keen to accept the responsibility of being independent practitioners, we need to be constructively critical of our own practices as well as those of others (Downe 1990).

## Professional organisations

Midwives have expressed their views through their professional organisations. The Association of Radical Midwives (ARM) and the Royal College of Midwives have both published policy documents: *The Vision* (Association of Radical Midwives 1986) and *Towards a Healthy Nation* (Royal College of Midwives 1987, 1991). Both publications advocated that the midwife be the first point of contact for the pregnant woman, and that the midwife should be the expert in the care of pregnant women in the absence of medical or obstetric complications.

## Continuity of care

Continuity of care is a big issue for women who have complained of seldom seeing the same midwife or doctor at antenatal visits. Women are no longer prepared to be the passive recipients of care and expect to be involved in the decisions about their own care. There are now numerous projects throughout the UK working towards continuity of care for women during pregnancy, birth and the postnatal period (Wraight et al 1993).

The 'Know Your Midwife' project (Flint et al, 1989) pioneered at St George's Hospital, Tooting, London, highlighted the problems faced by women seeing a variety of carers, and was the first time a large hospital unit in the UK had offered women-centred care. The most significant factor of the project was that the research was carried out by midwives and its publication brought the findings to the attention of the profession. Presentation of the study at the International Confederation of Midwives Congress in 1987 ensured a very wide audience.

## POWER, POLITICS AND CHANGES TO THE STRUCTURE OF THE HEALTH SERVICE

The latest, and probably most serious issue for women and midwives is the setting up of NHS Trust Hospitals on a national scale. By April 1994 over 90% of NHS hospitals had achieved 'Trust' status. Each hospital will be responsible for its own budget, selling its specialities to 'purchaser' health authorities and 'budget-holding' general practitioners. Although Trusts were designed to increase choice for consumers, block contracts are limiting purchasers to a narrow range of local options, and any referrals to other health authorities incur additional costs. Far from improving services, these measures will serve to limit the options of treatment offered by GPs to their patients and remove the choice of the place of delivery from parturient women.

## Conditions of employment

The other major concern is that 'Trust' hospitals are not bound to nationally agreed pay and conditions of service for staff. Each hospital can redesign contracts of employment by restructuring the service; staff can have their job descriptions redesigned; their existing contracts may be replaced, or they can all be given notice and invited to apply for newly created jobs en masse, with contracts of employment limited to 1 or 2 years.

### 'Gagging' clauses

Many establishments have also included a contractual clause inhibiting nursing staff from speaking out about particular policies, procedures and practices in the employing hospital. The threat of dismissal is a strong deterrent for potential 'whistleblowers' and despite promises to nurses, from the Minister for Health that no such 'gagging' clauses would be permitted, they are here. The UKCC Code of Professional Conduct requires that every registered nurse shall act at all times:

in such a manner as to justify public trust and confidence, to uphold and enhance the good standing and reputation of the profession, to serve the interests of society and above all to safeguard the interests of the individual patients and clients.

(Robinson 1986)

The two situations are completely incompatible and its is easy to envisage numbers of staff contemplating alternative careers where their moral standards are not compromised to such an extent.

### Pay

It took until 1988 for nurses and midwives to attain a living wage through clinical regrading, (although even now there are unresolved situations where staff are not paid in respect of their experience and expertise for the job they do). Once again all that was achieved is disappearing almost before it was begun.

There is a morality and myth in nursing and midwifery that the satisfaction of being involved in a 'caring profession' is sufficient unto itself and that financial remuneration is of no consequence, after all, nobody goes into one of these professions 'for the money'.

## A new hierarchy

Within the Trust system there is a new hierarchy with a Clinical Director leading the medical, nursing and midwifery services. To date these new positions have been almost exclusively the province of doctors, reinforcing the dominant–subordinate roles between the professions. Doctors have been able to exert more power than nurses in health politics; it has not always been to the benefit of the patient (Hand 1991).

Whilst creating a new management structure, elements of the old structure have been replaced, and it is the nursing and midwifery management that has been pared to the extent that some units no longer have directors of nursing or midwifery, or any senior managers beyond ward sister level.

### The multidisciplinary approach

In recent times progress had begun to be made through a multidisciplinary approach. The growth of the mutldisciplinary team concept has meant that nurses and other health care professionals not only expect but insist on being consulted and involved in decisions regarding patient care. While most doctors have tried to adapt to these changes, the notion persists among some that teamwork is merely a group of people doing what they say (Darbyshire 1987).

## EDUCATIONAL PROCESSES

All human beings are subject to inherent attitudes and are to varying degrees ageist, classist, homophobic and racists. Children's attitudes begin to form at a very early age and are reinforced by their nurturing environment, experience and education. Psychological processes do not always deal with the objective external reality that children actually encounter, but they are concerned with the internal reality: what all individuals subjectively make of the world they experience (Raphael-Leff 1991). Gender and social class have pronounced implications on the expectations of children and their abilities and opportunities to achieve. As children grow they are exposed to peer pressure, and religious, cultural and political factors which influence the development of attitudes. Given the complexity of the growth and development of these attitudes it becomes clear that changing attitudes of individuals or groups can be an enormous task.

At the sociocultural level, questions regarding the impact of gender and social class differences between physicians and nurses need to be raised. These differences could be seen as central factors in preventing conditions conducive to good communication (McLean 1988).

The lack of understanding between the professions begins with the separate educational processes of medical students and midwifery and nursing students. Although the training of nurses and midwives is no longer under the control of doctors, there is still a tendency for some lectures to be given by them. The reverse is seldom, if ever the case. In an American study of medical students' views of the role of the nurse, it was found that the students' perceptions of the physician's role vis-à-vis the patient and the health care team became more specific, while their perceptions of the nurse's role became more vague and diffuse. Medical students did not go to lectures by other health care professionals because students were not required to attend them, and were reluctant to spend their limited study time in classes that dealt with psychosocial aspects of health care (Webster 1985).

With new nursing education programmes being developed in universities and colleges of education, the subservient role is less evident and nursing students are entering the clinical field in a more assertive manner, and with a much greater awareness of research-based practice. Medical education also requires updating and changes are beginning. Already at King's College Hospital, London, medical students spend time working with nurses to gain a better understanding of exactly what it is they do, and a nurse tutor lectures them on the art of suturing (Hand 1991).

There is still a long way to go, but education is the key to a new philosophy. It is hoped that the changes which are still occurring will lead to a satisfactory model of care, as well as mutual respect between the professions (Wicker 1990).

For nurses who are teaching medical students in the clinical setting, timely advice on power games comes from a doctor who is herself grateful for the nursing contributions to her own education:

resist the temptation to humiliate them, since the intern (house officer) you belittle in 1985 could be the hostile doctor you have to deal with for decades to come.

(Ricks 1985)

## WHERE DO WE GO FROM HERE IN COOPERATION?

With all the historical factors in place and given the current situation in health care politics in Britain, it is hard to imagine any significant change in the balance of power for the foreseeable future. Doctors have it, and are unlikely to relinquish their hold, because from their point of view there is no political, financial or social advantage to a more democratic multidisciplinary approach. In all social change it is the oppressed and disadvantaged who advocate change. Doctors support each other and have a strong sense of professional fraternity. Too often, nurses appear to regard one another as rivals and adversaries rather than colleagues and partners (Editorial 1990).

It is also true that the nursing and midwifery professions reflect the low social status of their members; one example is that there is no mechanism by which the position and skills of a professional are recognised from one health district to another. A midwife may have been deemed competent to perform complex procedures and responsible duties in one area of the country, but once in another health district or even just another hospital in the same area, the same person may be inhibited from practising skills by hospital policies and by diffident managers with outmoded unproven habits. Midwives can find themselves in the unenviable position of accepting positions well below their clinical expertise and station, and hospital administrators have carte blanche to continue this situation in areas where there is not a shortage of staff or in Trust status hospitals.

In an effort to deal with this situation and to encourage continuing education among staff the English National Board has developed the Professional Portfolio for Higher Award. Basically it is designed to bring clinicians to degree level, and to show employers that the midwife/nurse has maintained her/his own education beyond the original training period. It is a good start but there is a necessity for a national recognition of skills and competencies as well as the existing registry of qualifications. If a police or fire officer is promoted his status is recognised anywhere in the UK; a transfer to another area would be to a job of the same grade and position, and the individual officer would not be expected to accept a lower position and salary. Perhaps the gender of the majority in these services has something to do with the arrangements. For nurses and midwives no such system exists. Blatantly political action has, in the past, done little to bring about changes. The quiet revolution through education and research would seem to be the path being taken by nurses and midwives to redress the balance. Medicine and nursing will remain two distinct professions, both with complexities, specialists and changing dimensions. Their areas of expertise are separate (Smoyak 1987).

For nurses and midwives it is crucial to maintain and expand communication with the medical profession. Dialogue is not capitulation and it is often the quiet voice of reason that prevails. There can be no end to hostilities until both parties feel exhausted from the perpetual antagonism. Once they admit fatigue, new avenues can be explored. Cooperation will lead to a greater understanding of each others' perspectives, to the benefit of the professionals, but above all to improve their individual contributions to the society they serve.

REFERENCES

Association of Radical Midwives 1986 The vision: proposals for the future of the maternity services. Association of Radical Midwives, Ormskirk, Lancashire

Darbyshire P 1987 The burden of history. Nursing Times

Donnison J 1988 Midwives and medical men – a history of the struggle for the control of childbirth. Historical Publications, London

Downe S 1990 Conflict of interests. Nursing Times 86 (47): 14

Editorial 1991 The doctor–nurse game. Nursing

Flint C, Poulengeris P, Grant A 1989, The 'Know Your Midwife' scheme – a randomised trial of continuity of care by a team of midwives. Midwifery 5(1): 11–16

Hand D 1991, Facts and fantasies. Nursing Standard 5 (17/19)

Inch S 1989, Birthrights: a parents' guide to modern childbirth. Green Print, The Merlin Press, London

Leap N 1992, The power of words. Nursing Times 88 (21): 60–61

Malby R 1989, Burying the hatchet Nursing Standard 3 (17)

McLean B 1988 Collaborative practice: a critical theory perspective. Research in Nursing and Health 11: 391–398

Morgan A P, McCann J M 1983, Nurse–physician relationships: the ongoing conflict. Nursing Administration Quarterly 7(4): 1–7

Peel Committee Report 1970 Domiciliary midwifery and maternity bed needs. HMSO, London

Pizurki H et al 1987 Women as providers of health care. World Health Organization, Geneva

Raphel-Leff J 1991 Psychological processes of childbearing. Chapman and Hall, London

Ricks A E 1985, What can you do now to make better doctors? RN: 36–37

Royal College of Midwives 1987 Towards a healthy nation – a policy for the maternity services. RCM, London

Royal College of Midwives 1991 Towards a healthy nation – a policy for the maternity services. RCM, London

Select Committee on Health 1992 Maternity services: second report of the House of Commons Health Committee (Chair Winterton N). HMSO, London

Smith L 1987 Doctors rule OK. Nursing Times 83(30)

Towler J, Bramall J 1986 Midwives in history and society. Croom Helm, London

Webster D 1985, Medical students' views of the nurse Nursing Research 34(5): 313–317
Wicker C P 1990, The nurse–doctor relationship. Nursing Times 86(4): 53
Wraight A, Ball J, Seccombe A, Stock J 1993 Mapping team midwifery. Institute of Manpower Studies, Brighton

# 14

# Comfortable men, uncomfortable women

*Tricia Murphy-Black*

## INTRODUCTION

The maternity services in the UK are undergoing a period of change which will have profound effects on childbearing women and may be decisive concerning the survival of the midwifery profession. This chapter examines some of the influences on the maternity services which produced a system of care designed for the comfort of the men who control the services, rather than for women they serve.

Walk down the high street of any British city and a variety of shoe shops will illustrate the title of this chapter. I have seen six such shops in one street in one city. The majority of these shoe shops are on two floors with the men's shoes displayed on the ground floor and women's and children's either up the stairs or down in the basement. A woman with a couple of children, perhaps one in a baby buggy, has a considerable struggle to get to the shoes she wants, for herself and her children. After buying the shoes, she has to negotiate the buggy, the children and her parcels up or down stairs to get back to the street. Lifts or escalators are rare. A man, probably unencumbered with children, walks in at ground level, chooses his shoes and walks out.

When I mentioned this to a number of mothers it evoked an immediate response; they had experienced exactly this situation. They also gave other examples of how difficult it is to take children outside the home: problems of getting on and off buses or trains; of going through narrow doors trying to hold children's hands; of pushing a buggy through a heavy door designed to swing back into place, and of finding women's toilets further away than men's. Leach in 1979 argued the need for a children-friendly environment in a children-friendly society. Has anything changed in the intervening years or do we in Britain still make life difficult for women with children?

Does this attitude, which is so prevalent in everyday life, also pervade the maternity services? Certainly the public rhetoric is that investment in the citizens of the future is a 'good thing'. Sometimes this general sense is used to raise public awareness and there are times when the maternity services, especially neonatal care, can use 'shroud-waving' very effectively to mobilise public resources. The development of the maternity services in the UK has been as chequered as that of any other service, and the subject of fluctuating opinions and fashions. The influences which have shaped these developments have had a variety of starting points. In asking if the maternity services are designed for the comfort of men while ignoring the comfort of the women they are supposed to serve, this chapter will examine some of these influences and demonstrate their effects on women and their babies.

## MATERNITY SERVICES IN THE UK

As the maternity services in the UK undergo the most radical reformation since the inception of the NHS in 1948, it has to be seen as a triumph for mothers. The word 'mothers' is used specifically, as it is the achievement of consumer power within one area of what is a male-dominated health service. Although women work in the health service, and indeed constitute the majority of its workers, they have not been as active in creating change within the maternity services as have the consumers. There are, of course, exceptions and a number of women working within the health service have campaigned actively for change, both with mothers and within their own organisations. The recent proposals to make the maternity services women-centred (Welsh

Office 1991, Department of Health 1993, Scottish Office Home and Health Department 1993), however, owe much of their impetus to childbearing women. It is both a sad reflection on the policy makers and those who interpret policy, and a matter for the congratulation of women that they have achieved such a shift in attitude and policy. Although the three policy documents differ in detail, the main message to emerge is pithily encapsulated in the title of an article by Page (1992): 'Choice, control and continuity'. Women have been denied both choice and control, for many years. There was little or no choice about becoming pregnant and once pregnant, even less choice. Even as recently as 100 years ago, the maternal mortality rate and death of babies, either during or shortly after birth, left little choice to women. Without choice, there was nothing to control. The wealthy might be able to obtain the best care available, but even that did not prevent tragedies. The poor had even less chance as they often started childbearing from a state of malnourishment and chronic ill health.

The rosy view of the 'golden age' of midwifery is that the local midwife provided continuity of care, not only through pregnancy and childbirth, but with each succeeding child. There may be some truth in this, but as Allison (1992) has made clear, the work of the district midwife involved a heavy caseload, and in order to survive midwives had to book a large number of mothers, which meant that the amount of time available for individuals would have been limited. She gave an example of two midwives working in geographical patches, who had a caseload of 233 mothers in a year. The midwives who worked this way nearly 50 years ago do not regret the changes in provision of midwifery care. The challenge today, however, is to be able to provide continuity of care without losing the employment gains of the midwives.

## Development of the maternity services

The forerunner of today's maternity services came about because of army recruitment for the Boer War (1899–1902). The poor physical health of the men, especially the large numbers who were unable to join the army, was attributed to poor feeding in infancy and childhood, combined with maternal ignorance and inadequate devotion to duty. This changed the political attitude to childbearing; it became the business of the state (Oakley 1986). Although both women and babies were dying in childbirth, it was the realisation of how healthy men could serve the country that turned individual tragedies into a matter for national concern.

An official report in 1917 (cited by Oakley 1986) commented on the infant mortality rate of that year. As the rate had been an improvement on previous years, the report noted that there would have been an additional 500 000 men available to fight in the First World War if the infant mortality rate had been as low for the previous 50 years as it had been in 1917. The conclusion has to be that national concern for mothers and babies had more to do with the provision of cannon fodder than with the welfare of members of society.

The early moves towards organising antenatal care on a national basis started at the turn of the century, but remained sporadic and with little firm foundation. Indeed the progress of the following years could also be questioned. Oakley (1986) reported from an interview with Dugald Baird in 1980, who had qualified in medicine in 1922 and had held the Chair of Obstetrics and Gynaecology in Aberdeen:

My maternal grandfather was [a] well known breeder of Clydesdale horses. By the time I was fourteen I was quite an expert on sex and reproduction. Mares received better attention in 1914 than some women today.

With the establishment of the National Health Service in 1948, antenatal care was more uniformly available at both local authority clinics in the community and the hospital clinics. The Peel Report (Standing Maternity and Midwifery Advisory Committee 1970), which recommended 100% hospital delivery, paved the way for the massive expansion of maternity beds, often in new hospitals. When the 1974 NHS reorganisation changed the system of providing care from three different authorities, the midwifery services became integrated. Previously midwives were either employed within the NHS and worked in hospital or they were employed within the municipal system and worked in the community.

Although this would appear to have offered an opportunity to create a seamless midwifery service, it was the increasing centralisation of care into large maternity hospitals which was the single most important influence on the increasing fragmentation of midwifery care. The medicalisation of pregnancy and childbirth had been taking place since the start of World War II. During the 1970s and 1980s this process had important effects on the social and emotional care offered to childbearing women, and was almost enough to cause the demise of the midwifery profession. It was the culmination of the influence of the medical men.

## MEDICAL MEN AND MIDWIVES

The title of Donnison's book *Midwives and Medical Men* (1988) has been deliberately changed here. The story of the man-midwife taking over in those births that needed instruments, those that needed knowledge and those that paid the best has been well documented. As early as 1760 midwives were warning against the effects of men-midwives. Mrs Elizabeth Nihell in *A Treatise on the Art of Midwifery* was already complaining about lack of patience that resulted in the breaking of membranes and using instruments to save time rather than wait for nature. Her statement:

I should not dispair of seeing a great he-fellow flourish a pap-spoon, or the public being enlightened by learned tracts and disputations, stuffed full of Greek or Latin technical terms, to prove, that water-gruel or scotch-porridge was a much more healthy aliment for new-born infants than the milk of the female breast, and that it was safer for a man to dandle a baby than for an insignificant woman'
(Nihell 1760, cited in Donnison 1988)

contained more prophecy than she could have imagined. The baby-milk companies may acknowledge the superiority of human milk, but as there is no profit to be obtained from it, concentrate their efforts on the 20th century equivalent of water-gruel or scotch-porridge.

Care by a man-midwife became fashionable and in order to enhance their importance, men-midwives emphasised the dangers of childbirth so that their attendance was seen as essential. Denigration of midwives' understanding and competence as well as blame, often unjust, was part of the armoury of the men-midwives used to increase the number of women who would want their services (Donnison 1988). These services, of course, cost more than those of the midwives so, that it was the well-to-do who were able to afford them. The poor, who would be less able to be generous towards the midwives, had no choice but to use a woman midwife.

Not only did men-midwives use their higher social status to be able to attend the better-off women but they also made an ally of the monthly nurse. By attending a case with a doctor the monthly nurse was able to gain financially. In those instances where a midwife was not employed, the nurse would not have to share the customary gifts with the other women attending the birth. Another bonus was that the man-midwife sometimes added a tip, so that the monthly nurse would encourage the employment of a man-midwife (Donnison 1988).

## The midwives' struggle for recognition

During the latter part of the 19th century, the struggle for recognition of midwives and for regulation of their practice had come to nothing, and the word 'midwife' was tainted with the image of Mrs Gamp (a drunken uneducated woman portrayed by Dickens). The very conditions into which midwives had been driven into by the men-midwives, who took the more lucrative cases, meant that they were forced to work long hours to survive and had little time for education or transmitting their knowledge in written form. Because of the trend towards an all-male, all-medical profession that controlled childbirth, women were not only deprived of a possible occupation but 'all women seeking skilled assistance in childbirth would henceforth be forced to put themselves into the hands of men' (Donnison 1988).

It was in the 1880s that those midwives who had managed to obtain some education, started the political battle against the situation where the rich were well provided for and the poor were dispossessed of midwives to provide care (Towler & Bramall 1986). In the struggle for education, a recognisable qualification and decent pay it was men again, albeit not only medical men, who opposed these moves. Objections, for example that the lower fees of midwives would deprive medical men of their income from obstetrics, or the proposed requirement for a certificate of good moral character, caused the failure of early attempts to have an Act of Parliament passed. Finally, after eight attempts in 11 years, the first Midwives' Act was passed in 1902 for England and Wales (Towler and Bramall 1986) with a corresponding Act in Scotland in 1915.

Training and regulation of practice, provided by the Central Midwives' Board (CMB), had been achieved through the Midwives' Act. Although the purpose of the Act was to provide training and regulation, and to prevent work by unqualified midwives, that is, to protect the mothers of the nation, it was argued that it also raised the status of midwives. This status was, of course, controlled, and that control was exercised by men. Even in previous centuries, the system of Episcopal licensing of midwives (Donnison 1988), which conferred the status of moral rectitude, was also designed as a means of social control.

The Central Midwives' Board had nine members, none of whom had to be midwives and only one of whom had to be a woman (although there were three midwives on the first Board). The chair of the CMB was a man and this position continued in male hands until 1973 when it had only 10 more years of existence. Towler & Bramall (1986), referring to the first CMB, give a clue to a more subtle form of control: 'Ironically, though, the member appointed by the Midwives' Institute had to be a doctor rather than a midwife'.

The Midwives' Institute (the forerunner of the Royal College of Midwives) had been active in campaigning for the Midwives' Act. The requirement that they, the professional organisation for midwives, had to appoint a member of the opposing profession was more than ironic. In addition two nurses' organisations also had the power of appointment. Midwives have never had complete control over their own profession, and this may explain some of the reduction of the profession's confidence in itself in the next 80–90 years.

## THE RISE OF THE EXPERT

Despite the midwives' struggles for recognition of their own professional status, they along with others, took on the role of expert in childbearing to combat what was seen as maternal ignorance; to teach the mothers so that they would produce good cannon fodder.

## Maternal ignorance

In the early 20th century, the UK suffered from the combined effects of a decline in birth rate and high infant and maternal mortality. As with so many social situations, the solutions arrived at were complex. In this instance, the solutions concerned not only the need to educate women, provide better food and improve working conditions, but they were also a response to the suffragette movement. Women who were occupied with the 'true' role of women (pregnancy, childbirth and child care, or to put it more cynically, pregnant, barefoot and in the kitchen) were not in a position to campaign for votes for women (Oakley 1986).

The aim of correcting maternal ignorance had already been taken up by the lady sanitary inspectors. In the 1860s the Ladies Health Society of Manchester and Salford had been set up for this very purpose. This group later developed into the health visiting profession. The original patronising approach of the 'Ladies', the 'do-gooders', continued for many years by reputation if not in fact, and this reputation was extended to the mothercraft classes which for many years were aimed at teaching mothers good hygiene

The creation of the public attitude that childbearing was the concern of the state removed it from the private and placed it in the public arena. The increased understanding of the physiology of childbirth combined with the technological explosion of the latter half of this century has turned the normal life event of pregnancy into an event which had to be submitted to the hands of the expert. At the same time as removing the confidence of women in their own bodies and experiences, the expert has become the controller.

## Midwifery ignorance

Midwives have suffered, as have all women through the centuries, from problems in obtaining the education they needed. Unable to acquire the basic skills for recording and documenting their knowledge, they passed it on from one to another by example and by word-of-mouth. Those midwives who did write could only reach the few who could read (Donnison 1988).

Aware of this problem, Rosalind Paget, one of the early and influential members of the Midwives' Institute, set up lectures, a library and a journal for midwives (Cowell & Wainwright 1981). Since then there have been many midwives who have worked to improve the education of other midwives. The training has grown and developed from the original course of a few lectures to the degree courses in midwifery, established in the UK in the late 1980s and the 1990s. This education gives midwives access to knowledge but, more importantly, develops skills of critical analysis so that knowledge can be used for the benefit of women.

Is such knowledge used to benefit women? Midwives have suffered from the expertise of the men-midwives who took their livelihoods and reputations (Donnison 1988). Sadly, women have also suffered from the expertise of midwives, just as the midwives suffered from the experts (Kirkham 1988). There is a danger that the knowledge held by midwives is used to control women rather than to empower them. This is a common reaction of a minority group under pressure; the groups turns on those lower in the pecking order. Yet, as the recent changes in policy concerning the maternity services in Britain have shown, the midwives' greatest supporter is, in fact, the consumer. We should be prepared to use whatever knowledge we have to encourage, support and build the confidence of the women we care for, as these women will in turn, empower the midwife who can provide the choice, control and continuity women want.

## Female conspiracy

Midwives have also been drawn into the female conspiracy, where women conspire against women. At its most extreme this has been seen in other parts of the world where, for example, it was women, often the mothers, who actually undertook female circumcision and Chinese foot binding (Shorter 1982). While these examples have to be to viewed in the context of their time and culture, when economic dependence and the need to survive drove the women to follow such traditions, the pattern has been repeated by women in different times and cultures.

That women control other women by colluding with men, whether implicitly or explicitly, has been demonstrated time and again in the maternity hospitals of this country (Kirkham 1988). Once women have been removed from their own homes and have to submit to the rules of an institution, they lose their ability to use their own resources to cope with the physiological process of childbirth. Once again, women (midwives) have betrayed women (mothers), not with the physical harm of female circumcision, but perhaps in a way that will leave just as lasting psychological scars. The really sad aspect of this is that it is often done in the name of 'being a good midwife' that is, blindly following the rules designed for the smooth running of an institution rather than the needs of an individual.

## Women as victims

Not only have women had to survive at the hands of the expert, whether the medical men or the midwives, but they have long been placed in the position of victims, so much so that there is a popular phrase 'a mother's place is in the wrong'. While woman were blamed for lack of competence as mothers at the turn of century (Oakley 1986), the women's groups of the 1920s and 1930s who suggested that poor health and the maternal mortality rates might be due to poverty were ignored (Lewis 1990). The answer was not to remove the cause but to put women in the hands of men in hospital where their disease could be controlled.

Much of the victimisation of women has been subtle, such as the hidden history of the impact of disease on women. The rituals and the taboos which forbade the examination of women stemmed from the combined fears of the strength of female power and the jealous guarding of a man's property (Shorter 1982). Even such traditions as the churching after childbirth were double-edged. Some of its origins were in the thankfulness of surviving the risks of childbirth, but the other aspect was that women were unclean, dirty, and unwholesome and had to be cleansed before returning to society (Shorter 1982). A group thus stigmatised is victimised. The medicalisation of childbirth, intended to reduce mortality of the vulnerable, was a mixed blessing.

## MEDICALISATION AND HOSPITALISATION

The single most important influence on childbearing women and on the midwifery profession has been the increasing medicalisation and hospitalisation of pregnant women. Until and including the period between the First and Second World Wars, the main service for women was the provision of midwives to conduct home births. Hospital care, under the supervision of specialists, was available for the specific purposes of teaching and for those mothers who were considered in need of specialist care (Lewis 1990).

The point about the teaching (the doctors' need) as opposed to the specialist care (the mother's need) has been reiterated by Donnison (1988); that is the establishment of lying-in hospitals was due to an initiative by the medical men. This was to provide a regular supply of 'clinical material' to advance their own knowledge and to teach.

This helped to establish the 'sick role' of pregnant women. The medical men and their students only saw the women who had complications; their lack of experience of the normal process contributed to the argument that pregnancy was something which required expert, professional control. A medical man who did appreciate the normal process, such as Dick-Reed, had to struggle for an audience for his ideas of natural childbirth, and these were never fully accepted by the medical establishment.

## The move to hospital care

The proportion of women who gave birth to their babies at home remained high until the Second World War. Women evacuated during the war, unable to be in their own homes, accepted the idea of going into an institution for childbirth. Even so, the home birth rate in 1946 was 54% (Mugford & stilwell 1986). In the early postwar years, there were not enough hospital beds for all women to have hospital care; only those who fulfilled certain criteria (complication of pregnancy, previous poor obstetric history, primigravida or grand multiparity) would be admitted. The Association for the Improvement of Maternity Services (AIMS), founded in 1961, had the initial purpose of campaigning for adequate health care facilities for those who needed it (Mugford & stilwell 1986). The wholesale move to hospital care started after the Peel Report (Standing Maternity and Midwifery Advisory Committee 1970) which recommended 100% hospital deliveries.

This report was the most influential in the reduction of home births. The change from home to hospital was not the only effect, the other was of centralisation of services. This resulted in the closure of small hospitals throughout the UK. This was particularly relevant in Scotland, where the geographical spread of the population meant there had been many small GP maternity units (Scottish Home and Health Department 1980). The number of maternity beds in Scotland decreased by 580 to 2099 between 1981 and 1990 (Chaplin 1984, 1991). The proportion of GP obstetric beds fell steadily form 21% in 1977 (Scottish Home and Health Department 1980) to 9.2% in 1987 (Chaplin 1988) but then there was a relative increase to 11.1% in 1990, because of the reduction in consultant hospital beds.

These changes in bed provision have taken place despite an overall increase of 3000 births a year between 1977 and 1985

(Scottish Home and Health Department 1988). The result has been increased 'patient' turnover in maternity care, in larger and fewer hospitals. Such examples were repeated in other parts of the UK.

## Fragmentation of care

When over half the births were at home, the full range of midwifery care was provided by community midwives; that is by most of the midwives. The proportion of midwives working in hospitals increased as the number of hospital births increased.

This resulted in a change from holistic care to increased fragmentation of care: the diminishing of the role went hand in hand with increased specialisation. Robinson (1989), using data from a number of sources, demonstrated that in 1968 approximately one-quarter of hospital midwives in Britain were working solely on one aspect of maternity care and by 1979 this proportion had risen to two-thirds.

For the women attending the hospital throughout the child-bearing year, this meant that they were in contact with a wide variety of midwives as well as numerous other staff, prior to transfer home for care by the community midwives. By the 1980s, care provided by one or two known midwives was rare.

## Design of hospitals

Hospital design also had its impact. The old hospitals had wards to provide both antenatal and postnatal care each with its attached labour rooms. Although cut off from the community, there was some continuity of care from the hospital midwives. In planning of the new maternity hospitals, the labour wards were centralised to provide a range of services and specialised equipment. The staff became specialists.

Some parts of hospitals were specifically designed to facilitate the rapid throughput of women. For instance, in clinics the consulting areas were double-sided so that the obstetrician could examine one woman while on the other side of partition another woman was being ushered in and placed in the proper position for the laying on of hands. Apart from the complaints of being treated like cattle in a market (Rantzen 1982), the double cubicles meant that privacy was impossible.

## Consequences

The impact of medicalisation of pregnancy was threefold: on the obstetricians, on the mothers, and on the midwives. By the 1980s obstetricians were in control of childbearing women. The aim was good: the reduction of maternal and perinatal mortality. In striving for this laudable aim, the pendulum had swung too far; physical care was predominant so that the emotional and psychological aspects were not given their rightful place (Mugford & stilwell 1986).

The acceptance of their expertise, the 'toys for the boys', that is, the technological machines and the structure of the service (both design and organisation) put obstetricians at the centre. The argument for this centralisation is economic and powerful. The obstetrician who has his marked parking space, who probably only lives 10 minutes away (Mugford & stilwell 1986), who has all the equipment and staff he needs on site, becomes the pivot so that best use can be made of his expensive time. The closure of small uneconomic units reduces overall revenue costs. A system, however, which seems to exist to serve the consultant obstetrician is pervaded by an attitude which is at variance with that of service to the childbearing woman and her family. Centralisation is convenient and comfortable for men.

For the mother, heavily pregnant and struggling to get children on and off cross-town buses, centralisation is a less attractive option. There is a catalogue of justifiable complaints, for instance: the 'cattle market hospital clinics', mentioned earlier' (Rantzen 1982); unacceptable waiting times in antenatal clinics (Boyd & Sellers 1982); too much intervention in labour (Prince & Adams 1978); conflicting advice (Farley's Report 1988), and routinised and impersonal care (Smith 1981). This selection of summaries merely reflects a persistent trend to be found locally and nationally, of women begging that the maternity services care for the whole woman and not just her gravid abdomen.

That other female group in the maternity services, the midwives, have also suffered from the medicalisation of pregnancy. Socialized not only into the structure of a place for the sick, and its strict hierarchy, uniforms and rules, but also trained within the sickness model, the midwife of the 1970s and 1980s emerged with a picture of care which was sharply compartmentalised, specialised and fragmented. Midwives, whatever their original ambitions or aims, were in danger of losing sight of the focus of their care, the women, and turning their energies to maintaining the smooth running of the institution. The consequences for midwives were a devaluing of their position with childbearing women. They lost their ability to provide a full range of care for normal pregnancy and birth. This development had a far-reaching impact on the self-confidence of midwives and the type of care available for women, with knock-on effects on the training and education of the midwives of the future (Robinson 1989).

## Honorary men

Of course, it will be said that not all doctors, not all obstetricians, are male. The proportion of females entering medicine is increasing but this is a recent trend. In the early days, female doctors suffered from problems similar to those of midwives in trying to assert their position. Have female obstetricians suffered from the same need to bind with their own group as have midwives? Have they adopted male attitudes as a result? Not only will they have had to be better than men to be accepted into medical school, but they probably have had to work harder to maintain that position. What does this do to their attitudes towards their own position and the position of the women in their care? Two personal anecdotes, one recent, the other nearly half a century old, may demonstrate this position.

The recent example is of a group of medical students, both male and female, striding down the corridor of a maternity unit, pushing open both sides of double fire doors, which have windows to allow those on the other side to be seen, and walking on without acknowledging that the door had hit me. That is unimportant, but as I had been standing at the entrance to the scanning department it could have been a pregnant woman. The rapid socialisation of new members to a group has been demonstrated by Melia (1987) and the lack of sensitivity to the needs of those they will be serving after qualification may have been picked up from their role models.

The other example concerns my own mother. She had been one of only two medical students in her year during the 1930s. Immediately after World War 2, after active service she was pregnant for the first time aged 35 so she decided (at 36 weeks gestation) to book for antenatal care. As my parents were living in

Scotland, where she did not know individuals, she asked for the names of the best obstetricians. Both first and second recommendations were fully booked for the following month. As the third recommendation was a woman, she decided to return to Ireland where she knew she would have the attentions of the best (male) obstetrician. When I heard this story, I asked why and her response was that she would not trust herself to a woman. She did, however, expect others to trust themselves to her (female) care. This example of double standards, I feel, is a demonstration of the 'honorary man' syndrome. The ones who lose out are not those who are the honorary men but the women for whom they care.

## THE RISE OF THE CONSUMER

During the last 50 years there have been established a number of lay organisations with an interest in childbirth. Although these have been founded with different focuses, their impact on the maternity services has grown in the last decade. The first was the National Childbirth Trust which started in 1956 to provide education and support for women who wanted an active birth. The campaign for improved health facilities by AIMS commenced 5 years later. The Maternity Alliance established in 1980, grouped together a number of organisations whose aim was to lobby for better maternity services and social benefits (Mugford & Stilwell, 1986)

In different ways, these organisations and others have had their influence on the maternity services. Sometimes acting as pressure groups; sometimes providing a focus for consumer concern over issues such as the sharp rise in the level of induction of labour in the 1970s; campaigning for active birth, and supporting the feminist obstetrician, Wendy Savage; these groups have had an impact on the maternity services (Kitzinger 1990).

Despite this success, these organisations, often small and frequently underfunded, have had to struggle against the antagonism of the professionals. Given the theme of this chapter, a report describing the paternalism of obstetricians would not be surprising. Sadly, however, midwives' relationships with women involved in these voluntary organisations has not always been supportive. Although the National Childbirth Trust, for instance, numbered midwives among its early teachers and this trend has continued, there were many years where the NCT spent time and effort teaching women how to defuse the antagonism of midwives who considered them cranks (Kitzinger 1990). It is to the credit of these bodies that they have managed to put consumer satisfaction on the agenda of the maternity services (Mugford & stilwell 1986) and that they operate very effectively on Maternity Services Liaison Committees.

## SISTERS SIDE BY SIDE?

The feminist movement may have changed the view of childbearing and rearing from the natural lot of women to something that should be controllable. Women, however, do not form a cohesive group and different views, attitudes and social conditions have their impact. Midwives are as varied as any other group, but in the interests of their own professional survival, they need to be clear about their purpose. Once midwives have the confidence to assert themselves as a profession dedicated to the care of women going through a normal physiological process, they will be able to fulfil their true function. Midwives should be 'with women', rather than with doctors, with fetal monitors, with biophysical profiles or with the demands of a clinic (Black 1982).

### Language

The language used by midwives can reveal the distance between them and the mothers they serve. Oakley (a sociologist) in the Social Support and Pregnancy Outcome Study (Oakley 1990) quotes from a comment by a midwife. Next to the word 'lady' there is a number referring to a note at the end of the chapter: 'The midwives referred to the women in the study as their "ladies"'.

This use of the word must have struck a sociologist sufficiently that she had to explain why it was there although she does not comment. Why are women called 'ladies'; is it a gesture of respect? It is better than calling them 'girls', but to my ears has a certain condescension. I wonder if midwives would describe themselves as ladies? How do midwives react when obstetricians refer to them as 'girls', or even worse, as 'my girls'. Protesting about this, whether within the formal context of meetings or more informally is not easy. The response can be derision against feminists or dismissal by saying that it is only meant to be friendly. Yet the obstetricians would not like to be called 'my boys' by a midwife.

Kirkham (1983) in her study of interactions between midwives and mothers in labour described the limited information provided as 'verbal asepsis'. The most striking word in the examples used is the word 'just'. Much of the information is limited by saying 'I'm just going to do . . .'

Another example is the use of language which surrounds vaginal examination. I have often heard midwives say 'the doctor is going to give you an internal'. As it is a procedure, and an uncomfortable one at that, it is probably a gift few women would want to accept. The most noticeable example of this difference was one where I was in a position to change it. The (then) Health Education Council asked me to comment on a draft version of *The Pregnancy Book*, designed to provide women with information about pregnancy and childbirth. References to the work of the midwife were unexceptional; 'the midwife will examine you', but it was the doctors who 'will give you an internal'. Discussion with the author resulted in keeping the language straightforward and untechnical but without the word 'give' in that context. Not only do midwives need to consider the language they use but also they need to pay attention to the consumer.

## Listening to the consumer

Discussion about the language of midwives may be of interest, but the focus on communication skills must not be confined to talking. There is a need for each of us to use our two ears twice as much as our one mouth.

Birth plans, which are now accepted as part of the normal planning of care, have been formalised, and become part of the standard form-filling. Yet, 20 years ago, such forms did not exist. A woman who wanted to control any of her childbirth experience, risked the wrath of the professionals, by asking for a list of requests to be attached to her case notes. Such case notes were immediately recognised, and the woman was classified as a troublemaker even before she had been met at the labour ward door. There was an assumption that whatever was requested would be impractical and that by building up such false expectations the woman was bound to be disappointed. It is one of the achievements of the consumer movement that birth plans have been so well accepted.

In the change from challenge to the staff, to something produced (therefore controlled) by the hospital staff, these plans may have lost some of their impetus. Part of individualised care is to be able to meet the needs of all women, and some women do not want to plan their birth experience. That said, the return of completed birth plans for the purposes of evaluation has been particularly low in one hospital (a rate of 12% over a year, Sargent 1994). This may indicate the completion of these forms in the early postnatal period has been of low priority rather than lack of interest. However, reports of midwives saying that the birth plan drawn up while attending one hospital has no relevance when the mother is transferred to another is not encouraging. It is remarks such as these which can turn the experience of birth into one which is remembered with horror and dread.

With the view of the consumer firmly on the political health care agenda the increasing collaboration between consumer groups and professional organisations is encouraging. The critical abilities of midwives need to be put to good use in challenging not only their own practice but also the accepted wisdom. The voices from the wilderness are beginning to be heard. In challenging the assumption that hospital is the safest place for birth (Tew 1990) it has been realised that much of the improvement in perinatal mortality can be attributed to the general rise standards of health and living conditions which have occurred in the past 50 years (Mugford & stilwell 1986).

Of course mothers want a safe delivery of their babies. In the vast majority of cases, this has been achieved and it has become the popular expectation. Stories passed between women, on the whole, do not include death of friends, neighbours and relations in childbirth. The very success of the maternity services has raised expectations so that mothers no longer focus on safety when expressing what they want from childbirth. They now expect, and rightly, to be able to start the new life with their baby with confidence, and having had a happy as well as safe pregnancy and birth. The most useful contribution of the midwife to this desire is to offer support.

## Support

For clinical and professional reasons as well any ideological reasons, as midwives we should put the support of women high in our priorities, whether this is support for a decision, such as a desire for a home birth, or providing the physical and emotional support needed in labour.

A study examining supportive activities in labour demonstrated that from 616 random observations, just under 10% of the nurses' time was spent in support. Supportive activities for this study were defined as emotional support, physical comfort measures, giving instruction/information and in advocacy (McNiven et al 1992).The study was undertaken in Canada (hence the reference to the nurses giving care in labour), and it would be interesting to see if there would be any increase in the amount of time spent in supportive activities if the research was replicated among midwives. This study had its limitations which the authors recognised, and although they would not generalise from the findings, they pointed out that the results were consistent with a previous randomised trial carried out by Hodnett & Obsburn (1989a,b).

Support during labour has been demonstrated as improving a number of maternal and neonatal outcomes, leading for instance to shorter labour, reduced neonatal complications (Klaus et al 1986), and improved interaction between mother and baby (Sosa et al 1980). An earlier Canadian study, where continuous, one-to-one professional support was provided during labour, showed that the experimental group had a reduced incidence of analgesia and anaesthesia use and episiotomies, and meant that the women exceeded their expectations of the level of personal control they would achieve (Hodnett & Osborn 1989a).

Support should not be considered an option.

Social and psychological support of pregnant women should be an integral part of all forms of care given during pregnancy and childbirth. Unfortunately it is not. The available data from relevant controlled trials suggest that penalties for ignoring these aspects of care can be expected not only in terms of psychological morbidity but also in less desirable health behaviour and avoidable physical morbidity in both women and their babies. ... No adverse effects of these forms of care have been reported, however, so they should be adopted forthwith so that more women and their babies begin to enjoy their beneficial effects.

(Elbourne et al 1989)

## CONSULTATION WITHIN THE HEALTH SERVICE

Massive changes have been taking place in the organisation of the health service in the UK in the last few years. The policy of decentralisation of management implemented by the Conservative Government has been well defended by its instigators and attacked by its opposers. By 1994 when most hospital services, and many community services have achieved 'Trust' status at different times during the last 4 years, some are in a position to evaluate the impact of self-governing status, while others are still in the midst of the early stages of change. The issue to be addressed here is not of effectiveness, but that of consultation with the public.

Once proposals to achieve Trust status had been accepted by the appropriate government department, the consultation phase began. Taking one such exercise as an example, glossy documents with details of the proposed changes were issued to health service staff and distributed widely to the public to serve as the basis for public consultation. The local Health Council (an organisation whose purpose is to represent the consumer view) produced summary versions of the larger documents which were sent, for instance, through the local government network down to the community councils (the lowest level of elected representatives), and set up public meetings. Despite this massive exercise, there was no question of keeping the hospital and community services under the control of the health authority. If this is the case, it has to be questioned why the consultation exercise was set up.

The numerous small maternity units, some free-standing GP units, some part of larger hospitals, that have closed in the last 10 to 20 years, did so despite the efforts of the women who appreciated the service they provided. As Martin (1990) has poignantly described, a survey of maternity services, funded on a shoestring, with 1107 women responding and worked on by the researchers in their spare time, was ignored in the decision making process and the closure of a much-loved maternity unit announced before the authorities has seen the results of the survey. Such actions produce a sense of futility, and raise questions like 'What is the point of marching behind banners, selling T-shirts and writing letters if the decisions are to be made by the comfortable men, ignoring the opinions of the uncomfortable women?'

## CONCLUSION

For many years, the Chair of Midwifery in Glasgow has been held by an obstetrician. The recent appointment of a midwife as Professor of Midwifery at the University of the Thames Valley has resulted in the present holder of the Glasgow Chair changing his title to Professor of Obstetrics (Page 1993). Is this a sign that midwives are making obstetricians feel uncomfortable?

Are women still uncomfortable within the maternity services and are men still the comfortable ones? Despite the uneven rate of progress, there is a shift in attitudes. The very success of the maternity services in reducing the appalling mortality figures of earlier centuries has meant that the expectations of parents are now different. Safety is still important, but the very assumption that pregnancy will have a successful outcome is a tribute to the achievement of the medical profession. The challenge now is that the focus needs to be on the structure and the process.

In the implementation of the recent reports in the UK (Welsh Office 1991, Department of Health 1993, Scottish Office Home and Health Department 1993), the centre of the maternity services had to be the childbearing woman and her family. Unlike Canada, where there is the advantage of starting midwifery services with a clean slate (see Tyson et al, Chapter 8) the British structure of midwifery services carries the burden of history. This structure includes the physical buildings, designed to fragment care, as well as the organisation of care. The ward- or department-based systems of care are being challenged by the setting up of teams or group practices of midwives, which aim to provide continuity of care, with a full range of midwifery care for women from a small number of midwives (Wraight et al 1993).

In this time of change to the structure, it is the process of care which needs attention. Early attempts to respond to consumer dissatisfaction were limited in some places to outward show, but pretty wallpaper in the labour ward does not make the experience of birth a satisfying one if the woman's expectations for choice, control and continuity have not been met.

REFERENCES

Allison J 1992 Midwives step out of the shadows. 1991 Sir William Power Memorial Lecture. Midwives Chronicle 105(1254): 167–174

Black T 1982 Are midwives 'with mothers'? Nursing Times 78(48): 2013

Boyd C, Sellers L 1982 The British way of birth. Pan Books, London

Chaplin N W (ed) 1984, 1989, 1991 The hospitals and health services year book, 1984, 1989, 1991. The Institute of Health Service Administrators, London

Cowell B, Wainwright D 1981 Behind the blue door. Baillière Tindall, London

Department of Health 1993 Changing childbirth Part 1. Report of the Expert Maternity Group. HMSO, London

Donnison J 1988 Midwives and medical men: a history of the struggle for control of childbirth. Historical Publications, London

Elbourne D, Oakley A, Chalmers I 1989 Social and psychological support during pregnancy. In: Chalmers I, Enkin M, Keirse M J N C (eds) Effective care in pregnancy and childbirth. Oxford University Press, vol 1

Farley's Report 1988 Is having babies the end of life as we know it? Crookes Healthcare.

Hodnett E D, Obsburn R W 1989a Effects of continuous intrapartum professional support on childbirth outcomes. Research in Nursing and Health 12: 289–297

Hodnett E, Obsburn R 1989b A randomised trial of the effects of monitrice support during labor: mothers' views two to four weeks postpartum. Birth 16(4): 177–183

Kirkham M 1988, A feminist perspective in midwifery In: Webb C (ed) Feminist practice in women's health care. John Wiley, Chichester

Kirkham M J 1983 Labouring in the dark: limitation of the giving of information to enable patients to orientate themselves to the likely events and time scale of labour. In: Wilson-Barnett J (ed) Nursing research: ten studies of patient care. John Wiley, Chichester

Kitzinger J 1990 Strategies of the early childbirth movement: a case study of the National Childbirth Trust. In: Garcia J, Kilpatrick R, Richards M (eds) The politics of maternity care. Clarendon Press, Oxford

Klaus M, Kennell J, Robertson S, Sosa R 1986, Effects of social support during parturition on maternal and infant morbidity. British Medical Journal 293: 585–687

Leach P 1979, Who cares? A new deal for mothers and their small children. Penguin Books, Middlesex

Lewis J 1990 Mothers and maternity policies in the twentieth century In: Garcia J, Kilpatrick R, Richards M (eds) The politics of maternity care: services for childbearing women in twentieth-century Britain. Clarendon Press, Oxford

McNiven P, Hodnett E, O'Brien-Pallas L L 1992 Supporting women in labor: a work sampling study of the activities of labor and delivery nurses. Birth 19(1): 3–9

Martin C 1990 How do you count maternal satisfaction? A user-commissioned survey of maternity services In: Robert H (ed) Women's health counts. Routledge, London

Melia K 1987 Learning and working: the occupational socialization of nurses. Tavistock Publications, London

Mugford M, Stilwell J 1986 Maternity services: how well have they done and could they do better? In: Harrision A, Gretton J (eds) Health care UK 1986 Burlington Press, Cambridge, p 53–64

Oakley A 1986 The captured womb: a history of the medical care of pregnant women. Basil Blackwell, Oxford

Oakley A 1990 Who's afraid of the randomised controlled trial? Some dilemmas of the scientific method and 'good' research practice. In: Roberts H (ed) Women's health counts. Routledge, London

Page L 1992 Choice, control and continuity: the three 'Cs'. Modern Midwife 2(4): 8–10

Page L 1993 Personal communication

Prince J, Adams M E 1978 Minds, mothers and midwives: the psychology of childbirth. Churchill Livingstone, Edinburgh

Rantzen E 1982 Introduction. In: Boyd C, Sellers L. The British way of birth. Pan Books, London

Robinson S 1989 The role of the midwife: opportunities and constraints. In: Chalmers I, Enkin M, Keirse M J N C (eds) Effective care in pregnancy and childbirth. Oxford University Press, vol 1.

Sargent E 1994 Personal communication

Scottish Home and Health Department 1980 Scottish Health Authorities' priorities for the eighties (SHAPE). Report by the Scottish Health Service Planning Council. HMSO, Edinburgh

Scottish Home and Health Department 1988 Scottish Health Authorities' review of priorities for the eighties and nineties (SHARPEN). Report by the Scottish Health Service Planning Council. HMSO, Edinburgh.

Scottish Office Home and Health Department 1993 Provision of maternity services in Scotland: a policy review. Health Policy and Public Health Directorate. HMSO, Edinburgh

Shorter E 1982 A history of women's bodies. Penguin Books, Middlesex

Smith L 1981 Diary of a postnatal patient. Clinical Forum, Nursing Mirror, 18th July, 30–31

Sosa R, Kennel J, Klaus M, Robertson S, Urrutia J 1980 The effects of a supportive companion on perinatal problems, length of labour and mother–infant interaction. New England Journal of Medicine 303: 597–600

Standing Maternity and Midwifery Advisory Committee 1970 Domiciliary midwifery and maternity bed needs (Chairman: J Peel). HMSO, London

Tew M 1990 Safer childbirth? A critical history of maternity care. Chapman and Hall, London

Towler J, Bramall J 1986 Midwives in history and society. Croom Helm, London

Welsh Office 1991, Protocol for investment in health gain – maternal and early childhood. Welsh Health Planning Forum. HMSO

Wraight A, Ball J, Seccombe A, Stock J 1993 Mapping team midwifery. Institute of Manpower Studies, Brighton

# Index